Gout Inflammation

Containing:

Gout Cookbook: Cooking With Spices

&

Anti Inflammation: The Essential Gout & Arthritis Meal Plan Guide

HR Research Alliance

D1534642

This one book contains two of the best selling books on the subject of gout & inflammation. We have put these two books together into one book. The information inside can really benefit someone who want to live a healthy lifestyle, and reduce inflammation through diet. Not just people who have Gout. But everyone can benefit from eating anti inflammatory foods. We thank you for ordering your copy, and would like to wish you all the best on your journey.

Thank you for ordering. Your reviews are greatly appreciated, and can help others who read them. Any knowledge you have based on your experiences, leave them in the review section of this book, to help out someone who can benefit from them. A small good deed such as that, can go a long way.

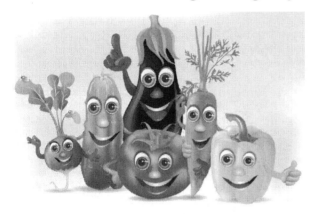

Join our newsletter & receive information on gout & inflammation. Links to our letter are inside of the eBook version of this book. Or, the free preview of the eBook on Amazon.

Table of Contents

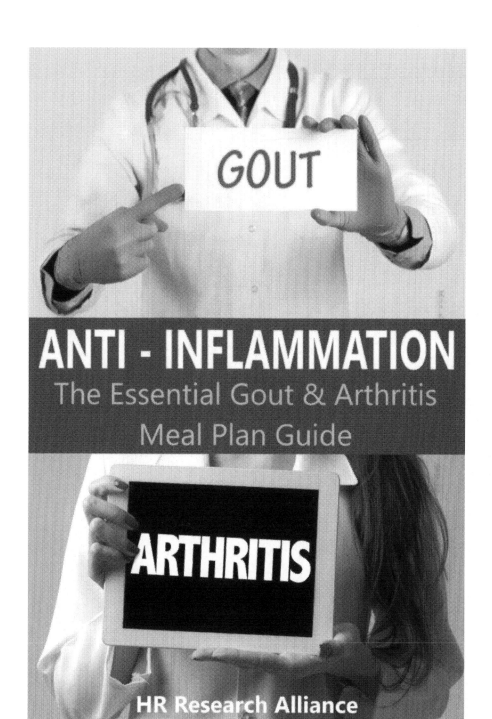

ANTI - INFLAMMATION
The Essential Gout & Arthritis
Meal Plan Guide

ARTHRITIS

HR Research Alliance

Anti - Inflammation

The Essential Gout & Arthritis Meal Plan Guide

HR Research Alliance

Nutrition is an essential part of life on earth. The body cannot function or survive with bad food, no food or water. Why is diet important? Here is what a balanced meal plan can do for gout and/or arthritis patients:

- manage symptoms
- cure or reverse some types of arthritis
- improve the quality of life
- protect the body and support its healing systems
- rebuild and repair damaged parts of the body
- help the body function properly by nourishing it

These are just a few of the benefits of quality nutrition and a healthy lifestyle. Although nutrition is not a universal cure, it is definitely a vital component in treating any disease, especially gout and arthritis.

The mere fact that dietary and lifestyle choices may stand at the root of these two conditions is proof enough that in order to get healthier, some adjustments need to be made.

The good news is these can all be controlled and achieved as long as there is an open mind attached to the will of living a happy, healthy, and long life.

The guidelines for managing these diseases are similar for the most part. The differences stand mainly in the types of foods consumed. The next lines discuss gout and arthritis as separate but combined conditions. At the end of it all, lifestyles will change and diets will improve just to prove the body is capable of much more when taken care of.

Gout & Arthritis - What do they have in common?

Arthritis is an inflammation of one or more joints. It is often accompanied by pain, stiffness, tumefaction, deformation or movement impair. This condition often gets triggered in the morning or after exercise. Arthritis is used to describe a group of over a hundred rheumatoid conditions that involve the joints. The most common forms of arthritis are osteoarthritis and rheumatoid arthritis. The following meal plan and dietary adjustments will discuss arthritis, in general, pointing to specific types of arthritis when required.

Gout is an acute form of inflammatory arthritis. Although both conditions are chronic diseases, meaning that they can't be cured, symptoms can be contained so as to slow down the damage to the joints. Gout is most common in overweight people or those with a diet based on saturated fats, a lot of food that is not so healthy and alcohol consumption. Gout affects the small joints in the hands and feet, especially the big toe; although it may extend to cartilages and other joints. Excess uric acid is responsible for developing gout. The uric acid crystals that have not been eliminated through urine build up in the joints and cartilages leading to gout attacks.

This condition may happen either because the body cannot properly excrete uric acid, it produces too much uric acid or there is an increased consumption of purine-rich foods. Purines are transformed into uric acid inside the body and may cause an excess that builds up in the joints.

The increased production of uric acid can be triggered by hemolytic conditions, an enzymatic deficit, psoriasis, Paget disease, alcohol, obesity or a faulty diet. Reduced excretion may be linked to renal disease, diabetes, high blood pressure, sarcoidosis, Down syndrome or diuretics. Causes may also be mixed, making it hard to establish one single culprit.

There is no way to tell for sure what causes arthritis. However, it's often regarded as the result of aging, diet or lifestyle. As with gout, arthritis is believed to have a genetic component. Being overweight does not cause arthritis but it definitely doubles the damage to the joints. This is why the first step with any treatment is to reach and maintain a healthy weight. It's no longer about looking better. It's about being healthy.

Another common feature is that they both lead to degeneration in the joints and an inflammatory response. What's more, they can both be prevented by adjusting the lifestyle and making changes to the diet. They are similar in symptoms: pain, redness, swelling in the joints. They disrupt inner balance and affect the quality of life. The lifestyle changes and diet for gout and arthritis are similar for the most part. In fact, there are certain changes that are always welcome no matter what the underlying condition really is.

Yes, these conditions are similar. One might say that gout is a form of arthritis, as mentioned in the beginning, which may be true, but there are so many conditions arthritis refers to that gout has separated itself from the group. Here is why:

Gout & Arthritis – What sets them apart?

A major difference between arthritis and gout is the following: gout is considered to be a metabolic disease, while arthritis is an autoimmune condition. What does this mean? It means that gout interferes with the way nutrients are broken down inside the body; it's more like a metabolic dysfunction, linked to the body's inability to properly function. Arthritis is the effect of the immune system's attack on healthy cells. The immune system regards the body's own cells, tissues as enemies and works towards destroying them.

In terms of causes and triggers, these two conditions differ for the most part. Arthritis is often generated by an injury or a genetic defect having to do with proteins found in cartilages. It can also be triggered by a bacterial, fungal or viral infection of the joint.

Although there is a lot of speculation to what causes arthritis, the truth is there is no way to know for sure. It's basically a mix of genetics and environmental triggers like a virus or bacteria. One thing is certain gout is caused by abundance of food and alcohol, which allows uric acid to build up in the joints. That being said, gout is caused by hyperuricemia.

Arthritis can affect any joint but it's most commonly known to affect the joints in the hands, wrists, and feet, whereas gout most commonly affects the big toe, knees and ankles. It also causes morning stiffness.

Gout always comes with redness, swelling and intense pain like the pain of giving birth. Fever has been noticed to come along with gout attacks. Arthritis may be painful but it doesn't always present with redness or swelling. The pain is associated with that of a toothache, although, there are times when the pain may be excruciating.

Gout affects more men. It starts affecting women after menopausal age. By contrast, arthritis affects more women than men and it's associated with old age (some exceptions apply, like juvenile arthritis).

A final distinction worth mentioning is the fact that gout can be prevented, while some types of arthritis can't. The genetic component is just too strong in some cases of arthritis that regardless of the lifestyle adjustments, healthy food choice, and practices, the disease still hits the body. Now, since this is too complicated to prove at the moment, the changes and adjustments needed for preventing gout apply to arthritis as well. It was to be expected given that arthritis is used to describe so many health conditions involving joint damage. But the distinction does not stop here. While arthritis may not be as preventable as gout, it can be reduced through proper treatment and even reversed. Not the same can be said about gout.

How to Treat Arthritis and Gout

Gout cannot be cured. Fortunately, it is highly manageable through proper medication and diet. Some forms of arthritis can be reversed. Given these two different outcomes, the treatment is basically the same for both. Why? Because both health conditions are somewhat similar in terms of symptoms and areas they cause damage to. Conventional treatment is first applied. Then dietary and overall lifestyle changes are a must in order to give the body a fighting chance.

Treatment is mainly symptomatic for both gout and arthritis. It works towards coping with pain and inflammation.

Treatment in arthritis differs depending on the type of arthritis. It mainly aims at:

- reducing pain
- lowering the inflammatory response
- preventing further deformation of the joints
- building bone structure
- reducing the frequency of flare-ups

- preserving overall health

Treatment of gout is anti-inflammatory, used to manage symptoms and correct the metabolic deficiencies. The next guidelines apply:

- relieving pain and preventing future gout flares
- reducing inflammation
- preventing damage to the kidneys and the formation of kidney stones
- reducing the production of uric acid in the body
- preventing further damage to the joints and the affected areas
- encouraging the body to properly eliminate uric acid

The medication prescribed for gout or arthritis is mainly anti-inflammatory. However, many of these drugs may present with side effects, one of which is nutrients depletion. It has been shown that arthritis patients have lower levels of folic acid, protein, and zinc inside the bloodstream compared to a healthy person. This may be due to medication which uses the body's resources to get to where it needs to. The body must work overtime. This is why a complete, healthy, balanced dietary approach is prescribed along with conventional medication.

Non-steroidal anti-inflammatory drugs and corticosteroids are used for managing gout and arthritis symptoms. Colchicine is often used to relieve pain and inflammation. Medication in gout works on four levels:

- reducing the amount of uric acid produced inside the body
- encouraging the kidneys to eliminate uric acid
- minimizing the frequency of flare-ups

- reducing the inflammatory response

The issue with medication is that it can have side effects when taken for a long period. A treatment strategy would be combining medication with alternative therapies that are not expensive and can be found right around the corner. There is no need to get fancy. It's all about small, simple, sustainable changes meant to become part of life.

Medication is not sufficient. Food has been used as medicine for a long time, in conjunction with what the doctor prescribes. Therefore, opting for a healthy diet plan associated with sensible lifestyle changes is the way to go. Leaving conventional medicine aside (drugs, surgery), what's left is nutrition along with supplementation.

Supplementing for Health

As noticed, a disease drains the body of nutrients, so does medication. Since there is no way around this situation, one must turn to additional help that may come in the form of supplements.

For the body to regain lost nutrients, it can turn to food or food supplements. There are a lot of nutritious foods, filled with beneficial substances that help fuel the body and restore its main functions.

Since both conditions present similar symptoms, the recommended supplements are basically the same. Some are more useful in arthritis as they also work on the immune system and others in gout for their effects on metabolic disorders.

Bromelain is a useful enzyme found in pineapples. It helps lower inflammation in both gout and arthritis. Pineapples need to be consumed fresh and juicy to reap all the benefits. If fresh pineapple is not handy, then bromelain supplements can do the trick. They are used to relieve pain in the joints, counter the inflammatory response, help manage arthritis and digest protein in the gastrointestinal tract. Taken in between meals, it helps to break down protein inside the body.

Essential fatty acids Omega-3's ease arthritis by suppressing the immune system's reaction towards its own components, working more like an anti-inflammatory. Stiffness in the joints can also be reduced by consuming fish oil, either liquid or pill form. Essential fatty acids (EPA & DHA) help control pain and the inflammatory response. Essential fatty acids can be grabbed from fish which is safe to consume in both gout and arthritis. They also help keep the nervous system healthy which is a plus.

Boswellia helps rebuild blood vessels around the inflamed connective tissues.

Olive leaf extract reduces the production of those agents responsible for inflammation. It can be used both in gout and arthritis to reduce inflammation and the associated pain.

Alfalfa contains a mix of important minerals. These present with various benefits for the human body. It helps facilitate the absorption of nutrients, such as calcium – great for bone health and proteins. It's available in powder form or as sprouts to use in a daily meal plan.

Sea cucumber is rich in specific lubricant substances found in joints and the synovial liquid. This one is particularly useful in arthritis.

MSM is an essential nutrient that helps reduce inflammation and contributes to repairing joint tissue. It's mostly recommended for arthritis.

Chondroitin sulfate and *glucosamine* supplements nourish the joints, ligaments, and tendons. They help build bones, ligaments, cartilages and synovial liquid in the joints.

Vitamin E is a powerful antioxidant that helps prevent free radicals from negatively affecting the joints. It has been shown to improve joint mobility.

Vitamin C is recommended on a daily basis. It can be supplemented without the fear of an overdose. It has a positive effect on the immune system and presents strong antioxidant properties.

Vitamin K helps deposit minerals in bones.

Brown algae supplements are rich in minerals that encourage bone health.

Calcium and *Magnesium* help prevent loss in bones. Minerals like zinc, copper, selenium should be added to the list. Selenium has antioxidant properties.

Vitamin B complex is helpful in inflammation as it increases the blood flow and reduces pain.

Niacin has a positive effect on arthritis patients; not so much in gout, where it should be avoided.

Folic acid supports metabolism and it is very useful in gout.

Shark cartilage helps reduce the symptoms of arthritis. It can also be used topically to relieve inflammation.

Garlic powder contains antioxidant substances and stimulates the immune system.

Corn silk contains proteins, fiber, carbs, vitamins, and minerals. It presents a diuretic effect and is helpful in both gout and arthritis.

Celery seed extract can be used to reduce inflammation.

Parsley used as tea may lower uric acid levels and counter the negative effects of gout and arthritis.

Other helpful plants that induce an anti-inflammatory state and soothe pain in arthritis and gout are devil's claw, cat's claw, burdock root, borage (starflower) oil, Cayenne pepper, noni juice, turmeric (Curcuma), and willow bark extract.

Minimizing Attacks/Flare-ups

Treatment of gout and arthritis is used to minimize the impact of flare-ups on the affected areas, stop the inflammatory process and prevent future attacks from taking place. During a gout attack, the best nutritional approach, setting aside drugs, is shifting attention towards fresh vegetables, fruits low in fructose, plenty of water and staying away from meats of all kinds for at least 1-2 weeks.

When considering remedies and treatments for any type of health condition, it's best to turn to a team of health professionals that can walk the body through a holistic approach. Long or short term treatment depends on the extent of damage to the joints and cartilages and the frequency of painful and inflammatory attacks.

Orthotics, braces, non-steroidal anti-inflammatory medication and plenty of rest is what the doctors prescribe. They also mention a better diet and plenty of moderate exercise. It's a great opportunity to put everything in order: losing weight and keeping it off, embracing a healthier approach to life and become better.

The strategy involved in minimizing attacks in both gout and arthritis is deciding what's best for the body and what makes it sick. It's all about understanding the implications of the disease, knowing what the treatment is, establishing dietary and lifestyle changes and sticking to them.

Gout & Arthritis Prevention

The great thing about gout and arthritis is that they can be prevented, most of the times. There are certain choices that influence the prevalence to suffer from one of these health conditions.

Prevention means bringing together those strategies that embrace healthy living and avoiding practices that may harm the body.

Risk Factors

The first step in a prevention program is to identify the risk factors. These are linked to either genetic factors or environmental conditions.

A genetic predisposition to suffer from a disease such as gout or arthritis is a risk factor. This does not mean that there is a 100% chance to suffer from gout or arthritis. Genetics combined with the same poor habits, disregard for good food and healthy practices will most definitely trigger symptoms.

Obesity is an underlying cause for most health conditions and it can exacerbate symptoms. Taking osteoarthritis and gout, for instance, excessive weight puts pressure on the joints leading to more damage and preventing the body from focusing on healing.

Smoking has been linked to rheumatoid arthritis. It's not sure whether smoking is one of the causes of arthritis but the fact that the absorption of nutrients is greatly hindered by this habit makes it unsuitable for arthritis patients. Calcium depletion is a contributing factor to destroying bones.

Next on the list is poor nutrition. This does not mean cheap food but food that only satisfies the taste buds and not the body's needs. The main culprits are sugars, saturated fats, alcohol in excess and large portions in one sitting. Going hungry for long periods of time may trigger an attack since it deepens the hormonal imbalance.

Dehydration is a risk factor. When cells inside the body do not receive the required amount of water, they start getting confused and no longer function as they should.

Prevention Strategies

Of course, it works to have a healthy lifestyle from the beginning, but for those not fortunate enough to share a passion for health, there are some strategies that can shift the body from sick to fairly healthy.

A prevention program focuses on eliminating all the risk factors that can be controlled. Once the risk factors eliminated, maintaining a healthy lifestyle is key to sustaining the results.

The strategies involved in preventing gout and arthritis are almost the same as lifestyle adjustments recommended for these two health conditions or for any other health issue.

Prevention strategies common for both gout and arthritis:

- *Paying attention to the quality of food –* nutrition is an essential, if not vital part of life; what goes inside the body shows on the outside sooner or later; fresh foods like fruits and vegetables support the body and provide valuable nutrients and fair amounts of water. A properly nourished body that gets the nutrients it needs on a daily basis is a body that will most likely be disease free. Staying high on nutrients like omega-3 fatty acids: fish oil, flax seed, fish, olives, coconut oil, nuts, and other seeds like chia; Vitamin D from sun exposure, fish, fortified whole grains, eggs or supplements during the cold season.

- *Reaching and maintaining a healthy weight* - losing weight too fast is no good; it, in fact, triggers more symptoms, more frequent attacks, and nutrient deficiencies that can make the disease worse. The body is in shock since it has to deal with all kinds of changes brought on by gout or arthritis. Submitting the body to another shock, like that of rapid weight loss, is not a good strategy. And it's not even sustainable. A smart way to lose weight is starting to listen to the body, understand that some foods are good and others not so much.

- *Regular exercise* can improve overall health and keep the joints and bone structure healthy. Non-impact exercises are recommended to reduce stress on the joints. Exercise helps with weight loss and helps build lean muscles to support the joints and improve the metabolic rate. Proper form is crucial, as well as adequate equipment.

- *Proper hydration* is as important as they say, dehydration being another risk factor.
- *Vitamin D* levels should never drop as they can hinder calcium production. *Vitamin C* is a great micro-nutrient used for its antioxidant properties and positive effects on the immune system.

Additional prevention ideas for arthritis:

- Quitting smoking is one of the best ways to eliminate one of the risk factors for developing arthritis. It can also help prevent other health conditions like cardiovascular and heart disease.
- High heels in excess have been linked to additional damage to the joints so no more for the ladies.

Additional prevention ideas for gout:

- Limiting meat consumption while increasing the amount of dairy has proven beneficial for gout patients.

- Purine-rich foods should be avoided (shellfish, organ meats).

A successful prevention program is based on small changes, one at a time, focusing on a stress-free body and mind. These two combined can make up worthy opponents for any health condition.

Diet Plan/Guide

A successful diet plan starts by establishing appropriate levels of nutrients needed by the body. This means knowing how much protein to eat, how many fats, carbs, vitamins, and minerals. Balancing macro and micro-nutrients is a sound approach to weight loss, preventing diseases and managing gout and arthritis symptoms.

Since weight loss might be an issue, the diet should be calorie-restricted but making sure not to go under the basal metabolic rate. Although the caloric intake is important to some extent, the quality of food is the one to have a major impact on the body. Food choices will be discussed later on.

The body needs to receive constant supplies of nutrients. This is why having around 5 meals a day is an excellent choice. In order to lose weight, the body needs to rest in between meals and allow hormones to function properly.

The body starts losing weight in 3 hours after a meal, provided that hunger does not become part of the equation. The key is finding nutritious foods that don't require large amounts in order to fuel the body for a long time. A distance of 3-4 hours between meals is recommended.

This also helps the body digest food and then focus on repairing damaged tissues, joints, and cartilages. Energy levels will stay up high and insulin resistance (associated with an increased chance of gout attacks) will not become a problem.

So, how much to eat? This depends on individual traits involving sex, age, activity, weight. A rough estimate would be between 1600 – 2000 kcal.

This meal plan guide focuses on foods to eat in gout, foods to eat in arthritis (be it foods that are simply allowed because they do no harm to the body or foods that can help reduce damage, minimize attacks and help relieve symptoms), foods to stay away from (either because they are generally bad or they are bad for gout or arthritis).

The diet guide does not stop here. It highlights the most beneficial supplements to use in gout and arthritis and it contains meal ideas for breakfast, lunch, dinner and snacks.

Now, it becomes a question of deciding whether the diet plan and lifestyle changes should be the same for both or whether there is a personalized solution involved. Since gout and arthritis present similar characteristics, some dietary approaches might suit them both but there are instances in which they differ completely (for instance, dairy is recommended in gout but not in arthritis).

A proper diet along with lifestyle adjustments may reverse some types of arthritis or even cure them, in some cases.

A healthy diet helps to:

- increase energy levels
- replenish depleted nutrients
- strengthen the immune system
- prevent further damage to the body
- reach and maintain a healthy weight
- protect overall health

It's not about major changes but simple, common sense lifestyle modifications may decrease inflammation and pain, while preventing further damage to the joints. A nutritious diet may also help rejuvenate the joints.

Foods to Avoid in Arthritis

There are foods out there that may contribute to getting arthritis or speed up its progression by increasing pain, inflammatory responses, and damaging the body's immune system or bone structure.

Some of the foods mentioned below may not be that harmful since it depends on each individual response. However, it's best to know potential enemies and keep a close eye on them.

Gluten is at the top of this list. Gluten intolerance manifests itself by causing allergies. This type of allergy may increase intestinal permeability. Gluten can be found in wheat, rye, barley and most packaged processed foods. When the body rejects gluten, the immune system starts attacking its own cells and tissues. Joint pain is one symptom so needless to say, gluten might just not work in arthritis.

Dairy is not recommended as part of a diet in arthritis due to casein, the main protein in milk and other dairy products. It can cause a great deal of pain for arthritis patients. Protein supplies can be restored by choosing other types of foods like legumes, seeds, spinach, and quinoa. However, dairy is rich in calcium, vitamin D, and probiotics (yogurt, kefir). If the pain does not get worse, then it's probably a good idea to consume low-fat dairy.

While on the subject, cheese is best avoided, as well as pizza, butter, and margarine. These contain high amounts of saturated fats that worsen the symptoms associated with arthritis and can predispose the body to other health conditions like high blood pressure, cholesterol, cardiovascular and heart disease. Red meat, in particular, should be eliminated or consumed in moderate amounts (once a week or once every two weeks). Saturated fats can also be found in desserts, cookies, pastries, and pasta dishes.

Trans fats are another horror story. These types of fats are dangerous for the human body. The body does not even recognize trans fats since they are artificial substances used mainly for preparing margarine, snacks (potato chips, puffs), fast foods, and most packaged baked goods. Since the body does not recognize trans fats, it gets confused and stores them as fat or as probable cause to develop arthritis or any other type of health condition.

Nightshade vegetables (potatoes, tomatoes, peppers, chili, and eggplants) are often mentioned as foods not to eat due to a substance in their composition called solanine. There is no clear evidence to support that these vegetables might increase pain in arthritis. However, some people have developed an excessive sensitivity to these foods that it's better to avoid them. It would be a shame to miss out on the nutrients nightshade vegetables contain so no sensitivity to them means more on the plate.

Sugar is slowly becoming the number one enemy not only to obesity but also to a healthy long prosper life. Sugar is responsible for hormonal imbalance, inflammation, cardiovascular disease and it is basically missing all nutrients. It brings nothing to the body but chaos and disease – consumed in excess of course. The occasional treat is not going to be abolished. Refined sugars and all those crazy sugar substitutes (high fructose corn syrup, rice syrup, glucose, maltodextrin, dextrose, sucrose to mention just a few) should be avoided. Here are some healthy alternatives: coconut sugar, honey, dates, or maple syrup. Bananas can also be used to sweeten things up a bit.

Vegetable oils like canola, sunflower, grape, corn contain Omega 6 which may trigger an inflammatory response so it is best to avoid foods that contain high amounts of this fatty acid.

Omega 6 can also be found in soy beans and some vegetables. It is not entirely bad for health but limiting the amount of these foods can have a positive effect on managing arthritis. These should also be avoided in gout.

Citrus fruits (oranges, grapefruits, lemons) are subject to controversy. Some people do not tolerate citrus fruits due to their acidic nature. However, these foods are nutrient packed and provide a lot of vitamin C. Their antioxidant properties propel them to the top. A sure way to know whether a food is good or not for an individual is by testing it for a month, noticing the effects of including or excluding a particular food from the diet. They help reduce inflammation and restart the immune system.

Fried and processed foods are bad. That's it. Nothing else left to say. Here is another useful tip while talking about cooking: Foods should not be heated repeatedly, grilled, fried or burnt.

Alcohol in excess damages the body. It starts by damaging the liver to the point it can no longer eliminate toxins. Hormones run wild when alcohol becomes present in the bloodstream and long behold here is the first sign of arthritis. Alcohol is particularly bad in gout since it may trigger painful attacks. Tobacco is mentioned as being a risk factor for developing arthritis or for increasing pain and inflammation by depleting the body of valuable nutrients, like calcium.

Sodium is responsible for keeping water inside the body. Water retention is a real problem and can lead to serious health issues. Increasing the amount of sodium in arthritis may determine an increased symptomatic response so more pain and inflammation. These are just some of the reasons for which lowering sodium intake is beneficial. Spices and herbs can be used to get more flavors to a dish instead of using salt, which more often than not gets used in excess.

Helpful Food Items for Arthritis

Although there is no proven way to prevent arthritis or a universally accepted diet plan to treat it, here is what to look for food wise:

- anti-inflammatory properties
- antioxidants
- healthy fatty acids (Omega 3)
- foods high in sulfur
- alkaline foods
- nutritious foods (emphasis on vitamins and minerals)

The main reason to change the current diet and lifestyle is to work towards minimizing damage to the joints. In order to achieve this, the diet for arthritis should contain healthy fresh fruits and vegetables, fiber, nuts, seeds, unprocessed whole foods, and alkaline foods.

Dietary changes in arthritis

An important approach is increasing the amount of foods that contain sulfur (eggs, onions, garlic, and asparagus). What sulfur does is help rebuild bone structures, cartilages, and connective tissues by increasing calcium absorption.

Fresh vegetables are great no matter what. Green leafy vegetables (kale, collard, turnip, Swiss chard, spinach, broccoli, romaine lettuce, cabbage, iceberg lettuce) contain fairly large amounts of vitamin K. Vitamin K is useful in arthritis due to its property to prevent calcium from building in arteries. It also contributes to strengthening the bones.

On the same page, fruits hold a special place. It's best to consume non-acidic fresh fruits, so less citrus fruits. Avocado is a great choice to also provide the body with healthy fats. Pineapple helps reduce inflammation due to bromelain, an enzyme found in fresh ripe pineapples.

Anti-inflammatory Foods

Celery is not for everybody but should become part of the diet for arthritis. It might have a taste that's too strong for some people to take in. This is why celery supplements have been invented. If no issues with the taste, then the root can be used as a garnish for meat, as part of creamy soup recipes or raw salads. Celery sticks may be combined with peanut butter or added in smoothies. Celery helps by reducing pain in the joints.

Ginger root can lower the inflammatory response in rheumatoid arthritis and osteoarthritis. Ginger plays an anti-inflammatory role in the diet. It is also a decent source of antioxidants. There might be issues having to do with its strong taste.

Nonetheless, it is totally worth it since it decreases the pain associated with arthritis. How can it be incorporated into a daily meal plan?

It can be consumed in supplement form, fresh over boiled or steamed vegetables, in smoothies, or as tea. It acts as an energy drink as well, leaving out the negative effects of a sugar rush. Ginger has the same positive effects on gout patients.

Turmeric is another great option for anti-inflammatory effects. It works by blocking inflammatory enzymes and can be beneficial in both gout and arthritis.

Cinnamon contains manganese, calcium, and fiber. Cinnamon is said to help in gout and arthritis by reducing symptoms. It can also help lower high blood pressure and cholesterol. It can be mixed with ginger and/or honey.

Capsaicin in cayenne pepper has analgesic properties, helping calm the pain in an arthritis or gout attack. This happens when the pain nerves are stimulated by this powerful substance.

Antioxidants

When thinking about fruits, the common thought should be all-in: cherries, strawberries, in fact, all types of berries, avocado, watermelon, grapes, apples, bananas. They all contain powerful vitamins and minerals the body can use to restore balance and focus on areas affected by arthritis.

Cherries seem to be the stars of a diet helpful in preventing and relieving symptoms. They are powerful antioxidants with anti-inflammatory properties due to their high content of anthocyanins.

Green tea can be used in rheumatoid arthritis and osteoarthritis as antioxidant and anti-inflammatory. It also contributes to weight loss so it's a win-win situation. Decaf green tea might be a better choice than regular green tea just because caffeine might increase the risk of arthritis.

Vitamin C is highly recommended as it supports the immune system and presents powerful antioxidant properties: peppers, peaches, strawberries, cherries, papaya, citrus fruits, kiwi fruit, black currant, Brussels sprouts, dark leafy greens, and tomatoes.

Healthy fatty acids

It seems that foods rich in Omega 3 are recommended no matter what. No wonder here since this fatty acid helps maintain overall health. Omega 3 is helpful in arthritis due to its anti-inflammatory properties. Omega 3 can be found in fish (salmon, sardines), seeds (chia, flax), nuts (walnuts, peanuts, Brazil nuts, cashews, and almonds), avocados, olives, safflower and olive oil. Oily fish (mackerel, trout, salmon, herring, sardines, anchovy, and tuna) is recommended twice a week, about 3-4 ounces. Cold-water fish has more concentrated amounts of Omega 3.

Nuts (almonds, walnuts, pine nuts, pistachios, cashews) are tasty, rich in healthy fatty acids, protein, potassium, calcium, magnesium, and zinc. Combining nuts with fruits helps reduce the insulin response and prevent hunger to set in prematurely. Nuts are good for weight loss and supporting the immune system.

Alkaline foods

Apple cider vinegar has an alkaline effect on the body which is always good for the joints. It also improves digestion.

Here are some other suggestions to increase the amount of alkaline foods: cucumber, kale, lettuce, pear, apple, bananas, berries, cantaloupe, chestnuts, spinach, onions, and beets.

Foods high in sulfur

Why sulfur? Sulfur is a trace mineral particularly known for its effect on joint health. It is good for hair, nails, and skin as well and supports the liver function. The following foods contain high levels of sulfur and should be included in a daily diet: asparagus, onion, garlic, eggs, fish, poultry, seafood, nuts, cranberries, and cruciferous vegetables.

To be on the safe side, a daily diet can also include MSM. MSM is a supplement that acts as a substitute for foods high in sulfur. It's often indicated as an adjuvant in arthritis to keep joints healthy.

Nutritious foods

The most important vitamins and minerals in arthritis are Vitamins B6 and B12, Vitamin C, Vitamin D, Calcium, Folic Acid, Magnesium, Selenium. Nutrient deficiencies may cause arthritis or make it worse. The same goes for gout.

Balanced amounts of vitamin D are known for contributing to arthritis prevention. Vitamin D is amazing for mood (which influences the outcome of any treatment or diet), bone structure and for slowing down the progression of osteoarthritis. Sunlight is the main source of vitamin D.

It does not contain vitamin D but helps the body produce it once it penetrates the skin layers. Since this is still the food category and vitamin D has been included here, it would be a good idea to mention some foods rich in vitamin D: cod liver oil, fish, eggs, mushrooms, and fortified whole grains are just a few examples.

A deficiency in vitamin D can lead to autoimmune diseases, a weakened immune system, and a shaky bone structure, among others.

Cruciferous vegetables help shield the joints and cartilages from the devastating effects of arthritis. They support the body's detox functions. Cruciferous vegetables (broccoli, Brussels sprouts, cabbage, kale, arugula, cauliflower, and collard greens) are rich in vitamin A, vitamin B complex, folic acid, vitamin C, manganese, magnesium, iron, fiber, protein, zinc, and Omega 3.

This is the best way to get more iron for the body to use. Iron should be mainly obtained through food and not with a multivitamin complex. Iron supplementation has been linked to pain, tumefaction, and damage in joints. This is why food should be the main source of iron intake.

Great iron sources are broccoli, Brussels sprouts, fish, cauliflower, green beans, peas, cabbage, and lima beans. Broccoli contains large amounts of calcium, vitamin K, and C. It can be used to prevent arthritis and slow down the progression of the disease (mostly useful in osteoarthritis).

Brown rice and oatmeal are the recommended grains along with amaranth, barley, buckwheat, bulgur, millet, whole oats, and quinoa. Quinoa contains high amounts of proteins and it can make for a tasty breakfast, lunch or snack. It can be combined with fruits, tossed in salads with spinach, arugula, endives, tofu, turkey or chicken. Foods high in histidines such as rice, wheat, and rye can be helpful, paying attention to wheat though due to its gluten content.

Dairy products can be substituted by almond, rice, soy or coconut milk. The supply of probiotics may come from other fermented foods like sauerkraut, kimchi, apple cider vinegar, kombucha, and pickled vegetables. These are great sources of healthy bacteria to support gut health.

Vegetable sources of protein (beans, lentils, soy) can successfully take the place of meat, at least once a day. Soybeans (tofu, edamame) are good choices as well but in limited quantities, since they contain phytoestrogens. It's safe for women at menopausal age since it can also replace the loss of estrogen and help fight arthritis.

Some beans contain all those minerals that the body is craving for in arthritis: zinc, magnesium, iron, potassium, folic acid. They are high in protein and fiber. The best way to consume them is next to a type of cereal or whole grain (red beans with brown rice, lentils with couscous).

Garlic might be one of the most mentioned foods to have all sorts of benefits on the human body. It brings extra flavor to the plate and generates a healing response inside the body. Garlic, onions, and leeks make up a fierce team that helps strengthen the body and prevent further damage to the joints, ligaments, tendons or cartilages.

Mushrooms are often disregarded or forgotten. They present with serious benefits in case of arthritis and gout. It's been thought that mushrooms may trigger attacks in gout or create an inflammatory reaction. The truth is that mushrooms actually contain beta-glucans, powerful anti-inflammatory carbohydrates. Mushrooms are a great source of protein, vitamin B and all sorts of minerals (manganese, zinc, selenium, phosphorus, potassium). They can be used in omelets, vegetable and meat dishes. They go great with parsley and/or dill. Adding garlic and olive oil increases their nutritional value.

Dark leafy vegetables, sweet potatoes, carrots, and squash represent safe choices for arthritis meals.

Note that fasting is not recommended in gout but rumor has it that it might help in rheumatoid arthritis. Although the effects wear off once the practice is stopped. This is worth mentioning since fasting has become somewhat famous.

Taking into account that arthritis is reversible the lifestyle and diet modifications might not need to be permanent. However, they are synonyms to ongoing health so why would anyone want to go back? The key to a healthy, balanced life is remembering that health slips away when the body is vulnerable. Most often, bad choices (be it food, drinks, work, the level of stress, activity, exercise) reflect on the immune system. A malfunctioning immune system is a perfect recipe for any disease to invade the body.

Foods to Avoid in Gout

It has been thought that a limited protein intake would help prevent gout; however, the new guidelines in the prevention of gout encourage avoiding fats and carbs. Not just any type of fats and carbs, but saturated fats and refined carbs. Fructose, sorbitol, xylitol and saturated fats have been linked to increased purine synthesis. Alcohol can also lower the kidneys' ability to eliminate uric acid making it bad for gout patients.

Arthritis and gout share some uninspired food choices, such as gluten, processed foods, trans fats, sugar, Omega 6 in excess, fried foods. Both require limiting sodium intake and alcohol restriction.

A healthy gout diet will eliminate most purine-rich foods, especially animal origin food items (organ meats and seafood). This is not necessary for arthritis, though saturated fats should be avoided in both health conditions.

Soft drinks and fruit juices should be avoided. A smoothie would be a better alternative. If it also contains at least one vegetable, even better. Fruit juices should be limited to once or twice a week, preferably diluted with water. Refined carbs determine insulin levels to rise and blood sugar levels to suddenly drop resulting in a spike of energy followed by a rapid burst of hunger and sluggishness. This means no more pastries, pies, white flour, sugar, candy.

Helpful Food Items in Gout

There are some food choices out there that help with gout symptoms. As mentioned, anti-inflammatory foods can be incorporated into the diet.

Dairy products are at the top of the list. Dairy has been shown to benefit gout patients by helping reduce uric acid levels. Dairy is not helpful in arthritis and is best limited. Gout patients can opt for low-fat dairy products and stick to them on a daily basis.

Citrus fruits are rich in antioxidants and should be consumed on a daily basis. They are rich in vitamin C and are just filled with energy. The consumption of citrus fruits is controversial in arthritis but one thing is for sure – it works wonders on gout (just because they are fun, tasty and juicy).

Low-fructose fruits are best for gout: plums, pineapple (beneficial in both gout and arthritis), berries, mango, apples, kiwi fruit, grapes, bananas, figs and so on. Fruits provide energy, vitamins, minerals, a little bit of fiber and antioxidants. Cherries are not good for arthritis only. They help reduce inflammation in gout as well and work their antioxidant effects.

Caffeine (not recommended in arthritis) may have positive effects on free radicals and help lower uric acid levels. Moderation is the key to almost every aspect of life, except for when one wants to be great (being great entails a little bit of excess, but it has to be a moderate excess of the good stuff).

As seen before, essential fatty acids are recommended in gout as well so in with nuts, fish, and seeds. Fish should be consumed once or twice a week.

Eggs are safe. This is great news since eggs can be used to create satiating breakfasts and much more. Potatoes are allowed in gout as they contain low amounts of purines.

A diet plan for gout contains foods that support kidney and liver function. These two organs are responsible for flushing out toxins so their role is vital, especially when they need to eliminate excess uric acid. Raw foods are responsible for triggering the body's detoxifying process. The following foods are good in gout and support liver function at the same time: beets, apples, broccoli, brown rice, onions, tomatoes, walnuts, turmeric, licorice, and cinnamon. Fresh fruits and vegetables help optimize kidney function: algae, bananas, celery, cucumber, papaya, parsley.

Meal Ideas for Arthritis

A meal plan for arthritis can be based on the Paleo diet, the Mediterranean diet, and a Gluten free diet. These three diets can provide excellent meal ideas and various sources of good food that can help ease arthritis. The trick is not to stick to just one but get the inspiration and concentrate it in great dishes that help the body.

The Paleo diet consists of eating meat, fruits, and vegetables, much like a caveman. Processed foods haven't been invented in a Paleo diet so no sign of them and cultivated grains are almost impossible to find. The only issue is red meat which should be limited.

This is why the Mediterranean diet comes along and suggests more fish, instead of red meat, more healthy oils to go with those fresh fruits and vegetables. The Mediterranean diet can be used to lower the inflammatory response.

A meal plan in arthritis can consist of 4-5 meals a day, at 3-4 hour intervals.

The next meal ideas have a little bit of everything – various foods combine and work together to repair and make the body stronger.

Breakfast

A good day starts with a healthy breakfast. As repetitive as this may be, it's true. Breakfast sets the body in motion and provides valuable energy. Breakfast should be tasty (as any food should) and satisfying. The day should start with a large glass of water about 15-20 minutes before eating. Most people complain about not having enough time to eat in the morning. Breakfast can be prepared the night before and consumed in the morning in just a few minutes. What's the next excuse?

Here are just a few ideas to make the most out of every morning:

- Baked squash with honey and cinnamon, nutmeg, cloves or cumin
- Boiled eggs on toast with baby spinach, tomatoes, and tofu
- Oatmeal with fruit, cinnamon, and chopped almonds
- Couscous with eggs, orange, peppers, tomatoes
- Flax and chia seeds pancake with almond milk

Lunch

The dietary approach in arthritis tends to be more on the vegan side. This is understandable since vegetables, fruits, plants, grains, and legumes are at the core of most healthy diets out there.

Lunch should provide energy for the rest of the day and comprise valuable nutrients (proteins, carbs, and fats):

- Raw vegetables with herbs and garlic yogurt dip (dill, chives, tomatoes, baby carrots, broccoli, cauliflower)
- Mixed salad: baby spinach, arugula, pumpkin seeds, cherries with Dijon mustard dressing (olive oil, apple cider vinegar, pepper, mustard)
- Bean salad with quinoa and zucchini stripes
- Cooked spinach with chicken and brown rice with a touch of turmeric and sesame seeds
- Brown rice with beans, avocado, and salsa

Snacks

Snacks play an important role in balancing hunger spikes and making sure more nutrients enter the body. It's basically another opportunity to enjoy good food:

- Cherry tomatoes with mozzarella and basil
- Banana dipped in chocolate sauce (a combination of coconut oil and cacao or carob) and rolled in coconut flakes
- Tuna sandwich with olives, cherry tomatoes, and lettuce
- Cherries and a glass of almond milk
- Oat cookies and sugar-free chia berry jam

Dinner

Meat should be consumed a few days a week (3-5 meals a week). It's a good idea to make 2-3 days meatless days. Of course, if meat poses no health issues, then it may be eaten as desired. There is no point in applying more stress to the body so if meat agrees with the body then it should not be left out that often. A light dinner is essential for a restful sleep:

- Mushrooms stuffed with vegetables and cottage cheese
- Salmon with lemon and herbs
- Oven baked chicken with fresh rosemary, garlic, and lemon
- Mixed vegetables, tomatoes, basil, garlic, oregano and salmon
- Bulgur with broccoli, mushrooms, and nuts

Meal Ideas for Gout

Gout has been linked to the Mediterranean diet so emphasis goes on healthy fatty acids. Apart from these, low-fructose fruits, foods low in purines, whole grains and dairy can provide some tasty meal ideas. The meals should strive to be complete, nutritionally speaking. This means that the meals should contain all nutrients the body requires.

There should be about 5 meals a day to avoid long periods without food. These might trigger a gout attack. Foods should be fresh as much as possible.

Breakfast

The following meals have been designed to boost the immune system, restore energy levels and prevent gout attacks:

- Pomegranate smoothie with bananas, yogurt and chia seeds
- Alfalfa smoothie from alfalfa powder and kefir
- Eggs with avocado, olives, lettuce, tomatoes
- Cottage cheese omelet with broccoli
- Scrambled eggs with spinach, mixed vegetables, parmesan and garlic

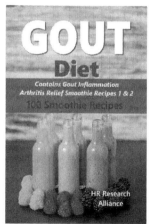 *Find great smoothie recipe ideas in this book. Order it on Amazon.*

Lunch

Be it at home, work, on the road or in between, lunch should be about enjoying a well-deserved break. The body stops at the nutrient station and absorbs good food. The trick is to listen to the body and give it what it needs and craves for. Maybe it's the following meal suggestions:

- Sweet potatoes with quinoa, turkey and raw cabbage salad with mustard dressing
- Brown rice, beans, green onion and mushrooms with goat cheese
- Lentils soup with vegetable rice
- Oven baked potatoes with herbs, served with salmon
- Chickpea salad with olives, quinoa, and fresh mixed vegetables

Snacks

Unlimited snacking may not be the case here since gout has a history with excessive eating. Nonetheless, choosing foods wisely and combining them efficiently may become part of a satisfying relationship with food for gout. There's nothing else left to say but enjoy:

- Mozzarella and grapes
- Yogurt with sesame seeds
- Green smoothie
- Red beans with salsa
- Buckwheat and kefir

Snacks should not be complicated. It's enough to use 2 or 3 ingredients to get great taste and valuable nutrients, plus it's easier to put them together or carry around.

Dinner

Here is where meat lovers can gather around the table and savor all those flavors that come along with a homemade meal or salad. Since meal planning for gout is related to a weight loss program, a sound approach would be that of consuming complex carbs in the first part of the day, leaving meat (poultry, fish) for dinner. The next step is adding in some vegetables and a homemade dressing. The last step is enjoying good food:

- Homemade chicken or turkey burgers wrapped in lettuce leaves with yogurt and olive oil dressing
- Stuffed eggplant baked with vegetables and chicken slices
- Fish with vegetables and lemon
- Chicken salad
- Roasted turkey with pineapple and sour cherry sauce

The trick to a successful plan that can be maintained for longer periods of time is paying attention to the body's response. No advantages come from eating bland food, foods that present no interest or foods eaten just because they are recommended for gout or arthritis. It's much more than that. This meal plan and the food ideas presented earlier are meant to propel the imagination and drive each individual holds to trigger a healthier start to life.

Lifestyle Adjustments and Changes to Manage Gout & Arthritis

Even though gout and arthritis may be genetic, this does not mean it is certain that either condition will actually manifest itself. Genetics combined with the same environmental conditions and the same lifestyle choices dictate the outcome. But what is a lifestyle? It is made up of every choice that influences one's life: food choice, sleep and rest hours, stress levels, work decisions, clothing, hair style, basically everything having to do with everyday life. No wonder that applying changes for the better can greatly influence the quality of life. This can also prove to be challenging.

Why Change?

Conventional treatment can't be used to solve every health problem completely. The good news is that gout and arthritis can be prevented through proper diet and other healthy lifestyle adjustments. Usually, what's good at preventing a disease, it's good for easing the symptoms in case it has already taken a toll on one's body.

Lifestyle changes for gout and arthritis may lead to:

- preventing gout and arthritis
- managing symptoms
- avoiding further damage to the joint and the body
- supporting healing as much as possible
- minimizing the frequency of attacks

Taking these benefits into account, there is nothing left than to find out what aspects of life to change and how.

Good Food to the Rescue

When adjusting one's lifestyle to better cope with health conditions, the first aspect to look at is nutrition. This includes knowing what foods to eat, what to avoid, understanding how the body interacts with food and how much it craves nutrients. There are foods out there that can even help treatment be more efficient and that support healing from the inside out.

A healthy diet is based on fresh food, home cooked from natural ingredients and no added sugars. More cooking may come in handy. Meal planning for a few days in advance can help save time and be prepared.

What does a healthy diet entail? It means eating fresh vegetables, fruits, whole grains, dairy, lean meat, nuts, fish, seeds, herbs. A healthy approach towards nutrition in health condition management means understanding what foods make matters worse and what foods help strengthen the body.

The More Water, the Better

It's recommended to avoid dehydration as this is the sure recipe for getting the body sick, triggering attacks and damaging the joints, cells, and tissues of the body. Water helps the body carry toxins out and contributes to an overall detox process.

Water is best consumed in between meals, starting the day with a glass full of water the moment that alarm clock goes off. The daily water intake should be of about 1 liter per 1000 kilocalories, so between 1.5 and 2.5 liters at least. These amounts go higher in the case of physical activity and climate. If drinking water does not come naturally, then adding fresh slices of cucumber or grapefruit can help make it tastier.

Supporting the Body through Sleep

Next on the list of lifestyle changes is sleep. The importance of sleep has long been debated and studied. The answer is experimenting and finding what suits the body best, as with food. The body knows what it needs to be healthy and keep on going for many years. When it sends signals like sleepiness, tiredness, sluggishness, the wise thing to do is listen to it and obey. This translates into more sleep and more leisure time. No worries, work will still be there.

Seven to eight hours of uninterrupted sleep a night is what the body needs to recharge its batteries and start the day fresh. Sleep allows the body to repair and focus on eliminating the damage done by gout or arthritis or any other disease. In arthritis, and during gout attacks, bed rest is recommended. The body should only focus on getting better and not on other types of activities.

Food may influence sleep as well so a healthier nutritional approach might solve any sleep issues that may cause additional damage to the body.

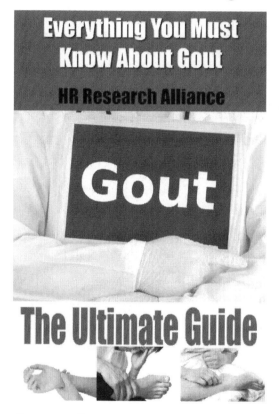

Great information on Gout inside of this book.

Regular Exercise Always Welcome

Regular exercise, properly performed with the help of a professional, is essential to keeping joint damage at bay. Here are some activity ideas to choose from: riding a bike, or a stationary bike, walking, swimming or water gymnastics. Contact sports and weight lifting might not be the best choices out there.

Tai chi is great for people of all ages and it's proven to be extremely helpful in arthritis as it helps strengthen the joints. Regular physical activity is great for a healthy body and a healthy mind to help cope with the symptoms of any health condition. Exercise helps with weight loss and maintaining a healthy weight. This change alone can improve the body's resistance to whatever may come its way. The idea is to get moving and not allowing the body to break down.

Outdoor activities are often recommended due to the increased oxygen amounts. It is also a great opportunity to get vitamin D levels to increase.

Managing Stress

Although many people know what stress is, it's hard to admit it as part of day-to-day life. Stress is a factor cumulus that disrupts inner harmony. The thing is stress often shadows every aspect of one's life. Stress leads to hormonal imbalance which further damages the body.

Staying out in the sun is a great approach to getting more vitamin D, elevate energy levels, and optimism. Since on the subject, Vitamin D is also used in bone formation. There are foods and activities that help manage stress. Green tea and ginseng are known for reducing cortisol levels (one of the stress hormones). Most antioxidants are helpful in lowering stress levels. What else lowers stress? A relaxing activity could be reading, listening to music, riding, yoga or meditation.

Losing the Extra Weight

Obesity has been linked to various health conditions, diseases and a weakening of the immune system. Losing the extra weight helps by eliminating the extra burden the joints must bear while struggling with gout or arthritis. Moreover, diabetes, cardiovascular and heart disease are connected to gout and arthritis and the link might be obesity.

The goal should be reaching a healthy, comfortable weight and maintaining it. The way to do this is by means of regular meals, not too much food in one sitting, no extreme hunger episodes, good and tasty food, leaving out those foods that are nutrient deficient and might have negative effects on the body. This does not mean letting go of every comfort food but finding balance and new, healthier ways to satisfy a craving.

Proper nutrition, adequate water intake, regular exercise, and good sleep represent the pillars of weight loss and disease management. It is not that easy but it basically is that easy once the goals are clear.

Other useful lifestyle changes:

- getting tested for food allergies (allergies have been shown to cause inflammation and may exacerbate the symptoms of arthritis)
- consuming less alcohol – alcohol in moderate amounts is not bad for the body; however, when the body is sick, it needs to be sober so alcohol should be limited or avoided altogether to allow the liver and kidneys to do their job properly
- increasing Vitamin C intake – Vitamin C is a powerful antioxidant that supports the immune system and the bone structure; it is recommended in a healthy environment as well just to be on the safe side
- choosing homemade foods rather than eating out – restaurant food might contain hidden ingredients (too much sugar, saturated fats or salt)
- giving meditation and relaxation techniques a chance

In order to be prepared, meal planning for a few days in advance might come in handy. It's best to consume fresh and organic foods but frozen foods may not be that nutrient depleted as thought. This is one lifestyle adjustment that can be implemented when suffering from gout or arthritis. Meal planning can help with weight loss as well.

Now, it becomes a matter of whether life is worth all this. Changing is not easy. What's important is to know the reasons behind the change and become aware of the satisfaction of the end result. If making adjustments to one's lifestyle means less pain, more energy, less stress, more health, this process is totally worth it.

To Sum Up

Gout and arthritis are related, there is no doubt about it. Some recommendations are common, others may differ but the main link between them is the desire to get better. When drive, meaning, and a specific realistic goal are present in one's life, everything comes together. Positive energy is a bite away. Food can nourish, comfort and help the healing process.

The purpose of a diet for any health condition is to:

- add more fruits and vegetables
- consume whole grains, legumes
- perform regular and moderate exercise
- consume no processed foods or chemically filled food items
- eat no refined sugars
- limit alcohol
- pay attention to a variety of foods

The guidelines are not written in stone. The approach should be that of trial and error by experimenting and noticing how the body reacts to stimuli, foods, and various practices that make up one's lifestyle.

Basically, a healthy, stable, balanced diet is required to be on the same page as getting better. Medical complications can be avoided by properly nourishing the body.

The main issue with any condition is the fact that the body becomes weak. When this happens, the body becomes the favorable ground for any type of condition to set in, such as heart disease or cardiovascular conditions.

The good news is that pain can be managed through medication, diet and lifestyle changes. Inflammation can be contained and joints can begin to repair. This happens when the body is properly nourished. And what better way to do this than by taking in every positive aspect of life on earth and incorporate it in day-to-day life.

It would be a shame not to take advantage of the opportunity to prevent or treat a health condition by making different choices. Nobody said it would be easy but having the proper tools and determination to get healthier means half-way there.

We thank you, and value your comments, and reviews for this book. Please share your experience with others, so they may benefit from your knowledge on the subject. Your experiences, and thoughts, can help benefit those struggling, more than you could possibly imagine. Placing your ideas, and experiences in the review section of this book, will make it seen by others, who will benefit from your help. 5 minutes of your time, can help change someone's life for the better. Thank you.

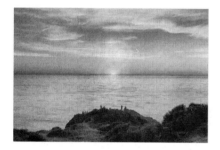

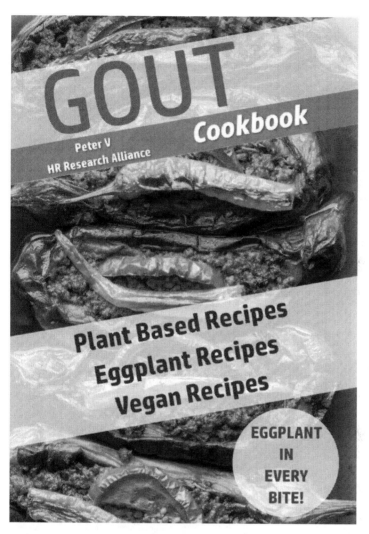

Looking for some healthy plant based recipes to add to your diet? Click this image and be directed to this book.

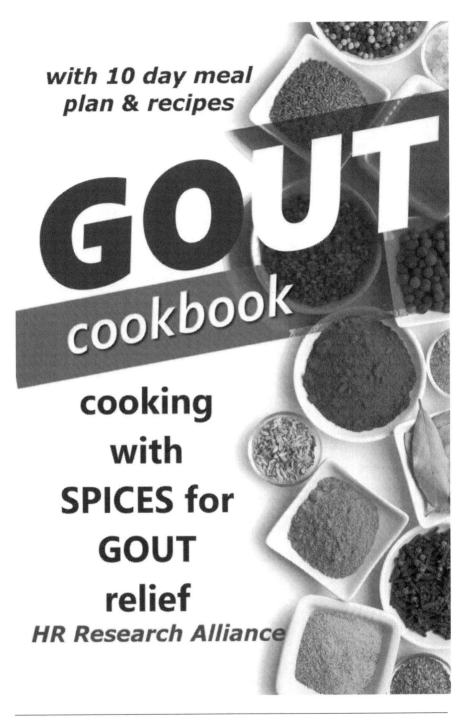

with 10 day meal plan & recipes

GOUT

cookbook

cooking
with
SPICES for
GOUT
relief

HR Research Alliance

Gout Cookbook

Cooking with Spices for Gout Relief

With 10 Day Meal Plan & Recipes

HR Research Alliance

Waking up to gout is frightening and painful. You went to bed fine the night before and you wake up one morning to an unimaginable pain. You may be suffering from just a swollen big toe, or you may have all over joint pain. However gout affects you, all you want is relief from the pain. While your doctor may have prescribed anti-inflammatories, there can be remedies right in the very foods that you eat to help you through this difficult time. Since they are food related, you may not even have to worry about food/drug interactions and may be able to use them side-by-side in your treatment plan. Just remember to talk to your doctor about any herbal or food related choices just to be safe!

Let's take a quick look at gout itself and then we will share some spices and other foods that help to bring relief and healing from a gout attack.

Gouty Arthritis Explained

Gout is a quick onset type of arthritis that hits you suddenly. Or so you may think. You see, when your first attack of gout hits the uric acid levels that cause the attack have been rising in your body for quite some time. Uric acid is a "by-product" of purine in the foods that you eat. Foods that contain purines include; cured meat, organ meat, dried legumes, beer, canned fish, and heavy gravies made from meat juices and fats. If you have risk factors for gout, your body is unable to break down and properly excrete purines via the kidneys and turns them into high levels of uric acid. HIgh levels of uric acid in your blood is called, hyperuricemia.

Gout pain comes from excessive levels of uric acid turning into crystals that settle in the soft tissues near the joints in your body. Most often, the first attack occurs in the joints surrounding your large or great toe.

Crystals rubbing on the joints and soft tissue leads to inflammation, swelling, and pain. Gout is often felt in the great toe, elbow joints, fingers, ankles, wrists, and knees. If gout continues untreated, the uric acid crystals may even build up and you may notice small bumps just under the skin around your joints and even in your earlobes. These bumps are known as, tophi. Uric acid crystals may also get stuck in your kidneys and form kidney stones. Tophi have also been found in the lungs and eyes. Because of these complications, early evaluation and treatment is very important. Gout tends to occur in "flares" and may last from days to even weeks. The flares tend to subside and go away, but may occur over and over again. Unlike rheumatoid arthritis where the symptoms are present on a daily basis, gout symptoms are only present during a flare. This may lead to a false sense of security that gout is gone and people may stop prevention and treatment measures thinking gout is no longer present.

The Four Gout Stages

Gout has a pattern and four distinct stages, although you may never know that you are in the first stage of gout. It is almost completely silent. The other stages are more pronounced. Once again it is important to know if you are at risk for gout, so you can begin preventative measures early on. Here are the stages:

Stage One: Silent or Asymptomatic Gout This stage is silently occurring right under your nose. There could never be a more perfect time to add healing spices to your diet. Look for things that help control uric acid levels and improve kidney function. This stage usually does not have any symptoms, but the uric acid levels are rising from the things that you eat.

Stage Two: Acute Gout Attack Stage two is actually the onset of a gout attack, with severe pain. Crystals from high uric acid levels are now damaging the soft tissues near and in your joints.

While you should see your doctor for evaluation and treatment, there are spices that may bring you relief during this intense stage of pain and inflammation. Spices may also help prevent a second or subsequent attack and shorten the course. Make sure to mention this to your doc.

Stage 3: Remission Period After the first acute flare subsides, you may be feeling great again! While the symptoms have gone away, you still are considered a gout sufferer. At this time, you will really want to "step up your game." You may not be in pain, but your body is still having a hard time controlling uric acid levels. This is another important time for preventative measures, like using spices that can control inflammation and uric acid in your cooking.

Final Stage: Chronic Gout Hopefully, you can reverse this stage with good care and preventative measures. Gout that is not fully treated can turn into chronic gout with recurrent attacks. If left untreated or undertreated, gout may cause permanent joint damage.

Gout Statistics

Gout is believed to affect more than 8 million people in the United States. Another 21 percent of the population has been found to have higher uric acid levels in their blood, putting them at risk for gout. If only they knew ways to manage this stage of the disease before it gets out of hand.

If you have risk factors for gout, it is a good idea to have your uric acid levels checked at your yearly physical. This way you can begin "gout prevention" measures to help ward off an attack. This could include eating foods made with spices that help keep uric acid and inflammation levels under control. This brings up the question, "what are the risk factors for gout?"

Risk Factors for Gout

The journey begins with knowing if you have risk factors for gout. Gout has multiple risk factors, the same as other types of arthritis. While a large portion of acquiring gout is due to poor diet, there is also a large underlying portion that is attributed to other things. These factors include:

- Alcohol Use (Beer)
- Diet High in Purines (Organ Meats, Gravies, Seafood, High Fructose)
- Family History of Gout
- Hypertension
- Diuretic Use
- Diabetes
- Obesity
- High Cholesterol
- Male Gender (Females are also at risk)
- Middle Age

One of the strongest of these factors is, obesity. Coupled with diabetes and hypertension can be a gold ticket to a gout flare. Obesity can increase the amount of pain you feel with attacks due to pressure on the affected joints. Obesity with the addition of high blood sugar can put a strain on the kidneys, reducing their ability to lower uric acid levels in the blood.

Symptoms of Gout

In order to get evaluated and begin early prevention in treatment, you should know the symptoms of a gout attack. This will help you recognize what is going on early in the game so you can take the steps to bring things under control. Symptoms of gout include:

- Joint Pain (Especially in the big toe)
- Pain and Discomfort in more than one joint
- Swelling, Inflammation and Heat
- Low-Grade Fevers
- Redness to the Skin
- Stiff Joints
- Itchy Skin
- Tophi aka Nodules under the skin near the affected joints
- Immobility

Any of these symptoms should be evaluated by a doctor as soon as possible. If you wake up in the morning with one swollen and red great toe with severe pain, seek medical attention that same day. This is a classic gout symptom with the onset of acute attacks.

Gout Diagnosis and Treatment

If you are at risk for gout, you can ask your doctor to check your uric acid levels at your yearly physical. This is important before you feel the pain of the first attack. You can start preventative measures right away and hopefully ward off an attack. Some preventative measures may include:

- Dietary Changes Eliminating High Purine Foods
- Reduction of Alcohol Use
- Increased Water Intake
- Increase Certain Spices in your Diet
- Exercise and Weight Loss
- Controlling Diabetes and Hypertension

If you are already suffering an initial acute attack of gout, your doctor will run necessary blood tests and possibly x-rays or an MRI to check the soft tissue near the joints. He or she may prescribe treatments to bring the attack under control. These may include:

- Anti-Inflammatory Medications
- Uric Acid Reducing Medications
- Diet Low in Purines
- Weight Loss
- Increased Exercise
- Extra Water Intake
- Rest Until Inflammation Subsides

20 Spices That May Relieve Gout

The good news is, when you have gout you have the option of many anti-inflammatory spices that can be included in your cooking to help relieve symptoms and lower uric acid levels. While you may be planning the foods you eat during mealtimes, what is equally important is the spices you use to cook your meals.

Dietary researchers have found that foods can cause inflammation in the body, or decrease inflammation in the body depending on the food. Some foods trigger your body to release chemicals that reduce inflammation, and some increase your body's production of prostaglandins, the chemicals that cause inflammation.

It is believed that if you add anti-inflammatory spices to your cooking, you can help prevent your body from releasing prostaglandins. People often don't realize that certain spices are very helpful in lowering inflammation levels in the body.

In any arthritis type condition, spices should be added to cooking throughout the day for steady and ongoing relief. Even starting with some cinnamon on oatmeal in the morning, curried soups for lunch, and ending the day with fresh basil tossed into a bowl of pasta at dinner. The spices may be minimal each meal, but the benefits add up over the course of the day.

Now that we know the best ways to use them in cooking, let's take a look at some of the top anti-inflammatory and pain relieving spices for gout relief:

1. Cinnamon

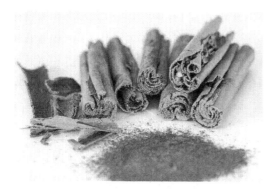

Cinnamon is a delicious and popular spice that can be used in both sweet and savory dishes for a spicy flavor. It contains cinnamic aldehyde and cinnamyl aldehydeis, which studies show these chemicals have anti-inflammatory properties. The effects are mild, but pack a good punch against inflammation when combined with another spice or food that has the same properties.

Try sprinkling some cinnamon on your hot or cold cereal in the morning. Use a dash in hot soups for lunch or dinner and use in hot beverages for extra flavor. The more often you use it during the day, the benefits will add up over time.

2. Garlic

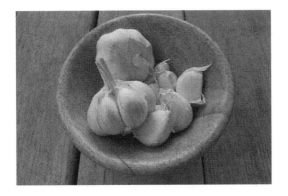

Garlic gives your food an amazing flavor and aroma, plus is versatile and can be used in any of your savory dishes. The anti-inflammatory chemical is diallyl disulfide, that reduces cytokines. Cytokines are one of the substances that increase inflammation in the body. Garlic is also a powerful antioxidant and has pain relieving properties.

The best way to eat garlic for its gout relieving properties is to use is freshly crushed into your foods. It is best crushed from raw cloves, as processed or dried garlic have weaker properties. Try some in your favorite pasta sauces, crushed over chicken before roasting, or stirred into hummus dip.

3. Cayenne Pepper

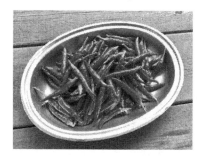

Cayenne peppers have a chemical known as, capsaicin. This has pain relieving properties by causing the body to release a chemical called, substance P. When the capsaicin enters the body or touches the skin it causes a slight burning sensation. Your body perceives this as pain and releases the substance P to signal the body to release its own pain relieving chemicals.

Cayenne is best in hispanic type foods, chili beans, and even rubbed on meats before cooking. You can also add a dash to potato salads or even soups. Always use it sparingly as it can be very spicy. Using it over the course of the day will help build-up pain relieving properties. You can also make a rub to use directly on your skin over the affected joints.

4. Turmeric

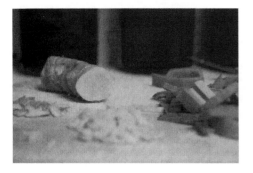

Turmeric is actually a root that contains a chemical known as, curcumin. This is a powerful anti-inflammatory that can actually block cytokines that cause inflammation. It also blocks other enzymes that cause inflammation in the body. It has been proven effective in several studies, with reduced swelling and pain in the joints.

Turmeric works best in Indian style foods and curries. Using it in combination with black pepper helps absorption. It will give foods a bright yellow color and adds a nice spicy touch to many different foods.

5. Ginger

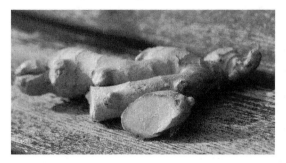

Ginger is a very popular remedy for many things including, inflammation. It contains both shogaol and gingerol that block the body's response to chemicals that cause inflammation. It may also have pain relieving benefits.

Ginger can be used in your savory foods as well as sweet foods. Use this root freshly chopped or ground for best results. You can even make it into a cup of tea with some honey and lemon. Ginger root may be effective for joint pain by making a paste and applying it directly to the skin over the affected joint.

6. Celery Seed

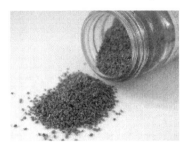

Celery seeds contain 3-n-Butylpthalidewhich, a potent diuretic that can increase the body's ability to flush out toxins like, uric acid. It makes your kidneys pull the uric acid from your blood and excrete it into your urine. It also helps to make your blood more alkaline. They have also been found to be rich in Omega 6 fatty acids and other powerful anti-inflammatory agents to help reduce inflammation and pain in the body.

Celery seeds can be sprinkled on salads or used in curry type dishes. It can be a very strong and bitter tasting spice, but used sparingly can add a nice touch to your spicy, savory dishes. You can also make it into a tea that you drink throughout the day.

7. Parsley

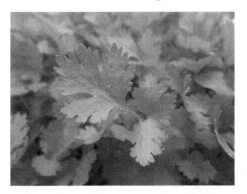

Parsley contains quercetin and kaempferol, which may help reduce levels of uric acid in the body. Parsley has natural diuretic properties to help your kidneys flush out toxins and may even help prevent kidney stones. It also contains a flavonoid known as, apigenin that reduces the body's ability to convert purines to uric acid.

Parsley has a wonderful bright natural flavor that can enhance any dish during cooking. It also makes a nice garnish that refreshes the breath and calms the stomach when chewed raw after meals.

8. Thyme

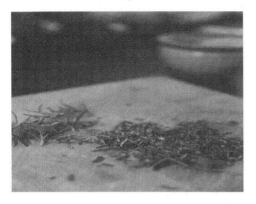

Thyme is another spice that contains high levels of, apigenin. This chemical can really help reduce the production of uric acid in the body from purines in the diet. Thyme also contains, carvacrol, which is a natural anti-inflammatory.

Thyme is good with chicken dishes, in soups, and stuffings used in poultry. You can also use thyme to make an effective tea for gout relief.

9. Basil

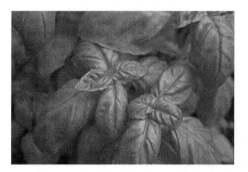

Basil contains a volatile oil called, eugenol. This chemical blocks cyclooxygenase or COX that increases inflammation during gout attacks. Eugenol works similar to NSAID's and pain relievers by blocking the action of COX.

Basil works great rubbed on meats, used in sauces, and even sprinkled in a salad.

10. Clove

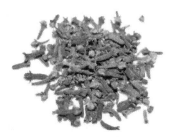

Cloves contain both apigenin and eugenol making them both helpful to lower uric acid levels and relieve inflammation. They are tasty in both sweet and savory foods when used in small amounts. They add a tasty twist to hams, spice cakes, spiked into an onion in stews, and steeped into a hot tea.

11. Coriander Seed/Cilantro

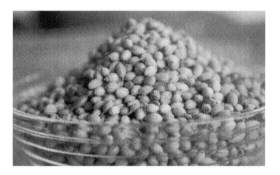

Coriander seed is actually the seed for the leafy green plant, cilantro. It contains two flavanoids, apigenin and rutin that were shown in small studies to help lower uric acid levels. It wasn't shown to have much of an anti-inflammatory effect, but can be paired with other spices that reduce inflammation.

Cilantro is a delicious addition to hispanic foods, salads, and side dishes. Coriander seed can be used as a thickener or spice in sauces and stews.

12. Lavender

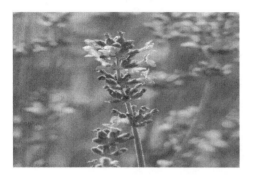

Lavender is showing signs of being a powerful anti-inflammatory. In studies that have been performed, lavender has almost the same effects as corticosteroids and prescription pain relievers. Researchers continue to look into why lavender has these effects, but the data seems very promising.

Lavender is delicious in sweet foods and desserts. It can also add an aromatic flavor to grilled shrimp, herb butter, and infused into sugar for cookies.

13. Lemon Balm

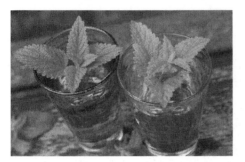

Lemon balm can have a powerful anti-inflammatory effect on the body. Two chemicals, rosmaric acid and quercetin both help lower inflammation in the body during gout attacks. Rosamric acid is also a very powerful antioxidant that may also help flush toxins out of the body like, uric acid.

Lemon balm is from the mint family and works deliciously in dessert foods, tossed into salads, and mixed into salad dressings.

14. Liquorice Root

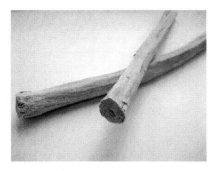

Liquorice has anti-inflammatory properties and may help relieve gout pain. It also helps block xanthine oxidase, the chemical in the body that turns purines into uric acid. Use caution with licorice because it can raise blood pressure. It is safe in small amounts.

15. Peppermint

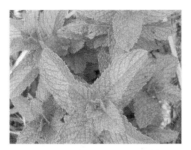

Peppermint is high in menthol oil that can help relieve gout pain. Drinking it in

tea may help reduce uric acid levels and you can rub a little on your inflamed joints for relief of inflammation and pain. Peppermint is a great seasoning for both sweet and savory dishes.

16. Rosemary

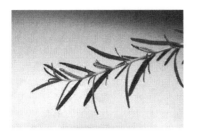

Rosemary is a strong and aromatic herb that can liven up the taste of any dish. Long used for gout, it increases circulation and helps the body get rid of uric acid. It can also reduce inflammation, redness, and the pain of gout.

Use some broken off twigs on freshly baked breads, sprinkle some in stews, or use as a garnish on hot foods. Heating rosemary will help to release the helpful oils into your foods.

17. Nettle

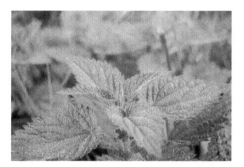

Stinging nettles may send a shiver through your spine when you think you might have to touch them. When harvested (with gloves, of course) they can be an amazing addition to things you cook. Nettle is a natural diuretic, increasing the kidneys ability to flush out uric acid from your blood.

Use garden gloves to harvest the leaves and rinse well. When you toss them into a pot of boiling water, the hairs are instantly neutralized. You may still see the hairs on the leaves, but the ability to sting is lost. Make sure you cook them well until the leaves are crisp. They work well to replace cooked spinach or even as a filler for vegetable lasagna. You can also toss it into stew, soups, or eat them sauteed.

19. Marjoram

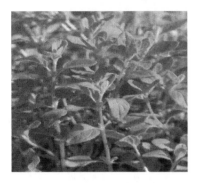

Marjoram has many different health benefits and can work as a pain reliever for joint and muscle pain. It can also help to relieve inflammation from gout. This spice also helps increase blood flow and helps to warm and soothe painful areas. The increased circulation encourages the body to clear out toxins and excess fluids. This effect may help reduce uric acid levels in the blood. It is encouraged to drink plenty of water when using marjoram.

Marjoram is a good seasoning to use in spaghetti sauce, tomato dishes, and on poultry. Make sure you use well chopped leaves and toss the stems out.

20. Fennel

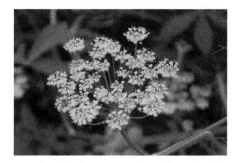

Fennel has natural diuretic properties and stimulates increased urination. It works first by helping remove uric acid from the body tissues and can help flush excess uric acid through the kidneys. By removing toxins, it can help decrease the inflammation in the body caused by gout.

Fennel has a sweet and licorice-like flavor, but it goes well in both sweet and savory dishes. You can use the entire plant, from the bulb to the leaves. Saute the bulb with onions and vegetables, sprinkle the leaves into a salad, or use leaves in sweet baked goods.

A Word of Caution with Spices for Gout

- Be sparing when you use a spice for the first time. Add a small amount and allow to simmer. Taste test after a few minutes then add a little more at a time. You really only need to start with a half-a-teaspoon, and work up to a full-teaspoon, if you desire. This is especially important if you are using a red pepper or cayenne based pepper. Cayenne really only needs to be added in "dashes."

- When using spices, try to find whatever you can fresh. Check the produce aisle to see if they have the spice available. If not, then look for a fresh chopped "jar version." As a last resort, it is okay to use the dehydrated version. Actually, some healthy antioxidants concentrate when dried and may be more powerful than fresh.

- Spices work well to compliment foods used as; rubs, liquid marinades, sprinkled on foods, tossed with pasta, used in soups/stews, or stirred into sauces. Since spices are "food grade" health supplements you can usually use any amounts you like, unless otherwise advised by your doctor.

Spices are mostly considered "low-purine" foods and most won't convert to or increase uric acid levels. There are some spices that may actually irritate and worsen gout. If you have high uric acid levels or are in an active phase of gout, you may want to avoid:

Poppy Seeds

Poppy seeds are extremely high in purines. They have about 170 mg per ½ cup. They are commonly used in baked items like; muffins, bread, bagels, and cakes. It is strongly advised not to use or eat poppy seeds with high uric acid levels or during an acute gout flare.

Sesame Seeds

Sesame is slightly lower in purines, but still over the recommended amount. Sesame seeds have around 60 mg of purines per ½ cup. They are commonly used in Asian and Middle Eastern foods. They can be used as an anti-inflammatory for arthritis sufferers, but it may trigger a gout flare. It is recommended to stay within moderate amounts if you choose to use sesame in cooking.

Pumpkin Spice

Pumpkin spice is the lowest purine containing spice, weighing in at only 44 mg per ½ cup. Since you may only use a few teaspoons, this spice may be okay. However, it is still advised to use this spice sparingly.

Recipes For Gout Relieving Foods Using Spices

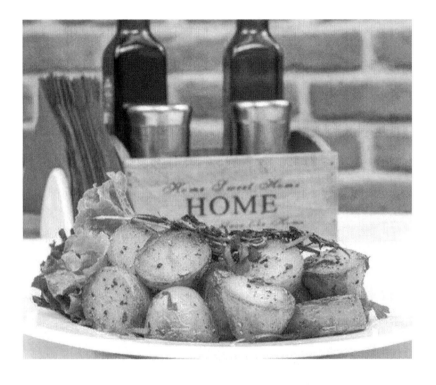

Using spices for gout relief can be easier than you think. These simple low-calorie recipes are quick to make with few ingredients for a busy lifestyle. Try these fast and easy meals to help relieve gout symptoms:

Soups and Starters

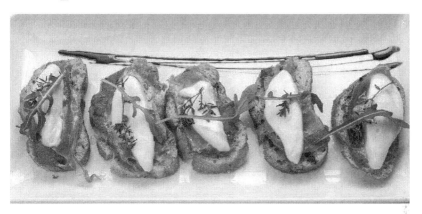

Kicking off a meal with a starter can awaken those taste buds and get them ready to taste the deliciousness of the main course. Starters can also calm hunger pains, while we wait for our meal to be ready. Some starters and soups are enough for a light meal or main course. Here are some helpful recipes to begin your mealtime, using spices that help alleviate gout symptoms.

Curried pumpkin carrot soup

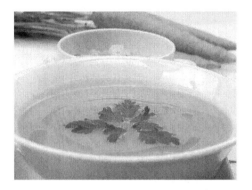

Soups can make a hearty meal that heals and warms your sore and aching joints. The flavor of this quick meal is both savory with a touch of sweetness. It pairs well with a chunk of crusty bread and good leftover the next day.

Ingredients

3 c.	**Pumpkin, Peeled and Cubed**
1 ½ c.	**Carrots, Peeled and Sliced**
1	**Potato, Peeled and cubed**
½	**Onion, Chopped**
½ c.	**Shallots, Chopped**
1 Tbsp.	**Ginger, Grated**

2 Tsp.	Curry Powder
2 Tsp.	Canola Oil
3 c.	Chicken Broth, Low-Sodium
½ Tsp.	Salt
¼ c.	Heavy Cream, if desired

Instructions

Heat Oil in large Skillet. Saute onion and shallots until tender and cooked. Pour in chicken broth and add potato, carrots, curry, and ginger. Simmer for 5 to 10 minutes. Add pumpkin and salt to taste. Cook 30 minutes until vegetables are soft. Use a whir blender to puree. You can add a dash of heavy cream at the very end of cooking if you like.

Stinging Nettle Pesto

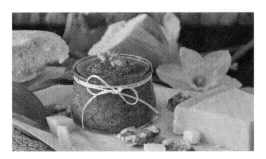

Pesto is a tart, nutty sauce that can be eaten on crusty bread, over pasta, or even as a marinade for chicken or fish. All the ingredients go straight into the blender and pulsed to the consistency you like. You can store any sauce in the fridge for up to a week and heat it up as needed.

Ingredients

6 c.	**Stinging Nettle, Raw and Packed**
½ c.	**Pine Nuts, Toasted**
2	**Garlic Cloves, Peeled**
1 c.	**Parmesan Cheese, Small Chunks or Grated**
3 Tbsp.	Lemon Juice

½ c.   **Extra Virgin Olive Oil**

Instructions

Throw Nettle, nuts, garlic, and cheese into blender and pulse until chopped well. Add in Lemon juice and olive oil in small batches and pulse. Continue to pulse until it reaches the consistency you like. Empty into pan and heat to use over pasta or place in a serving bowl to be used as a dip for bread or crackers. You can even use some over the top of steamed veggies.

Spring Mix Greens with Fennel Bulb

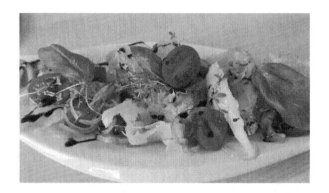

This light salad combines the sweet and crisp touches of spring mix greens and the "anise-like" flavor of fennel bulb. It works well as a first course or even with grilled chicken on top as a dinner salad. It only takes minute to toss up and works well with a vinegarette.

Ingredients

6 c.	**Spring Mix Greens**
3 Bulbs	**Fennel, chopped**
½ c.	**Cranberries, Dried**
1 Tbsp.	**Garlic, Minced**
3 Heads	**Radicchio, Chopped and Cored**

½	Purple Onion, Thinly Sliced
1 c.	Pecans or Walnuts
1 ¼ Tsp.	Sea Salt
¼ c.	Apple Cider Vinegar or Balsamic
¼ c.	Red Wine Vinegar
1 c.	Extra Virgin Olive Oil

Instructions

In a large bowl, mix together spring mix, radicchio, and fennel. Toss in cranberries and nuts. In medium size bowl, mix together olive oil, vinegar, salt, and garlic. Toss dressing with salad and top with a few berry tomatoes.

Pickled Cucumber Salad

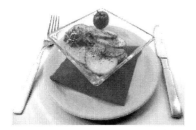

Cucumber salad can be a refreshing starter with your lunch or dinner. Most people will remember this on their grandmother preparing this light salad in the fridge. It really is as easy as she made it look and can be just as tasty.

Ingredients

3	**Cucumbers, Peeled and Sliced Thin**
¼ c.	**Sweet Onion, Chopped**
1 Tsp.	**Sea Salt**
¼ c.	**Sugar**
⅛ c.	**Water**
¼ c.	**White Vinegar or Apple Cider Vinegar**
½ Tsp.	**Celery Seed**

Instructions

Lay cucumbers out on paper towel and sprinkle with salt. Allow to rest for 40 minutes to 1 hour. Lay another paper towel over cucumbers and press down to squeeze out excess water. Place in large bowel. Sprinkle with celery seed and toss in onion.

In a separate bowl, stir together water, sugar, and vinegar. Pour over cucumber mixture and stir. Place in refrigerator to marinate for 1 hour.

Pico de Gallo Salsa

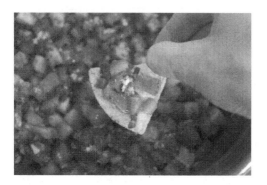

The key to the best salsa is, cilantro. Chopped into aromatic tasty bits and tossed with tomatoes, this can be a refreshing addition to any meal or great as a snack. It is good chopped up fresh or even the next day. You can use it on tacos, chips, as a marinade, or over some spicy enchiladas.

Ingredients

10-12	Roma Tomatoes, Diced
1	Sweet Onion, Chopped
2	Jalapeno Peppers, Cored and Seeded
1 Bunch	Cilantro
1	Lemon, Juiced
2 Cloves	Garlic, Crushed
1 Tsp.	Sea Salt

½ Tsp.   **Black Pepper**

Instructions

Dice Tomatoes and add to large bowl. Mix in chopped onion, chopped jalapeno, and cilantro. Sprinkle in salt, pepper, and garlic. Juice lemon into bowl and stir. Allow to sit for 20 to 30 minutes and then enjoy!

Main Dishes

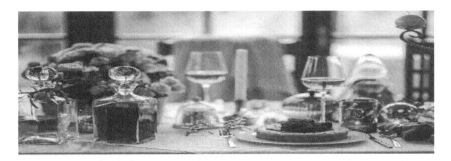

The main dish is the proverbial "star of the show," giving you the largest portion of the meal. These dishes were designed to be tasty, healthy, and satisfying. The use of spices make for some exciting flavor combinations when paired with sauteed fruits, vegetables, or sitting atop a bed of greens.

Pork Chops with Chopped Basil and Peaches

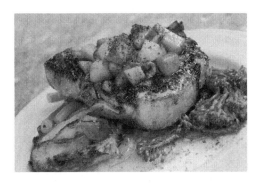

Wondering what to do with those pork chops? There are many exciting and tasty recipes for pork. Surprisingly, they work well with a number of spices! This recipe combines peaches, with fresh chopped basil to tantalize your taste buds and help with gout symptoms.

Ingredients

2- 4	Pork Chops
2 Tbsp.	Extra Virgin Olive Oil
3	Peaches, Cut and Pitted
2 Tsp.	Lemon Zest
2 Tbsp.	Lemon Juice
1 Tsp.	Sugar

½ Tsp.	Sea Salt
Pinch	Red Chili Flakes
2 c.	Spinach
1 Tbsp.	Butter
¼ c.	Basil, Fresh and Chopped Rough
¼ Tsp.	Black Pepper, Ground

Instructions

Sprinkle pork chops with salt and pepper. Heat olive oil in skillet and brown pork chops. Allow to sear 4 minutes on each side. Make sure internal temp reaches 145 degrees with meat thermometer. Take out of pan and set aside. Cover with foil. Add lemon zest, peaches, sugar, chili flakes and salt to drippings in skillet. Saute lightly about 3 to 5 minutes. Line plates with spinach and place pork chops over. Any juice that ran off pork chops onto holding plate, pour into skillet over the peaches. Add lemon juice and butter to skillet with peaches. Saute for another 3 to 5 minutes. Add basil and allow to reduce. Top pork chops with sauce from pan.

Coriander Chicken

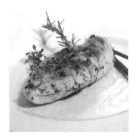

This tangy, spicy chicken recipe combines coriander with turmeric, and ginger. Three key spices that help with gout. It can be served up with couscous, risotto, or even steamed red potatoes on the side. The chicken can be cooked right away or place in the sauce to marinate overnight.

Ingredients

2 lbs.   Chicken Thighs or Breasts, Cubed

5-6 Cloves Garlic, Crushed

1 Tbsp.   Ginger, Peeled/Chopped

4 Tbsp.   Water

1 Tsp.   Coriander Seeds, Ground

1   Green Pepper, Seeded and Chopped

½ Tsp.   Cayenne Pepper

2 Tsp.   Cumin, Ground

½ Tsp.   **Turmeric Powdered**

1 Tsp.   **Sea Salt**

¼ c.   **Lemon Juice**

3 Tbsp.   **Olive Oil**

Instructions

Heat olive oil in skillet and brown chicken. Take out of pan and set aside. Place garlic into pan and saute. Add ginger and saute. Add in Turmeric, coriander, green chili, cayenne, cumin, and salt. Saute for 1 to 2 minutes. Place chicken into pan with water and lemon juice and simmer for 15 minutes. **Sauce as marinade:** In medium bowl, stir together olive oil, water, and lemon juice. Add garlic, ginger, salt, and spices. Place chicken in zip bag and pour marinade over. Place in fridge overnight. The next day, heat 3 Tbsp. Olive oil in pan and brown chicken. Remove chicken and set aside. Pour marinade out of bag and heat to boiling. Add chicken bag to pan and simmer until sauce is reduced. (Make sure sauce boils before eating to prevent food illness).

Glazed Ham with Clove

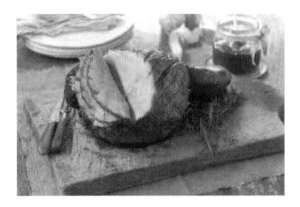

A glazed ham with clove can be a tender and succulent meal. A big enough piece of ham can give you leftovers for sandwiches, all while giving you the benefits of clove for gout relief. In this recipe, you will grind the clove powder and use it in the glaze. Making diagonal slices in the meat will allow the clove oil to both flavor the ham and infuse into the meat.

Ingredients

10 to 12 lb.	Ham, Boneless
¼ c.	Honey
1/2 c.	Brown Sugar
2 Tbsp.	Cloves, Ground
1 Tbsp.	Apple Cider Vinegar

Instructions

Preheat oven to 350 degrees.Take ham and make diagonal cuts about ¼ inch deep into meat, crisscrossing to form diamonds. Mix together; honey, brown sugar, clove powder, and vinegar in bowl. Use glazing brush to cover ham with glaze. If glaze is too thick, thin with orange juice 1 Tbsp. at a time.

Place in pan and cover with foil. Allow to roast for 1 hour. Open oven and carefully remove foil. Brush ham with glaze to coat again and cover with foil. Roast for 30 minutes and then spoon remaining glaze over the top. Leave foil off and turn oven up to 400 degrees and roast for a final 10 to 15 minutes until glaze is browned.

Chicken Tacos with Pico de Gallo

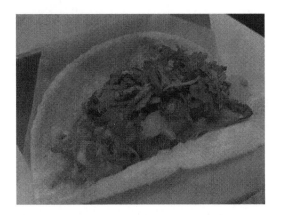

When you're craving mexican, chicken tacos spiced up with a little cayenne in the taco seasoning and topped with fresh pico de gallo is sure to satisfy. The chicken can be cooked up quickly that day, and salsa made the day before. Both the cayenne and the cilantro will help relieve gout symptoms and give your food that unique mexican flavor.

Ingredients

1 lb.   **Chicken Breasts, Boneless, Skinless**

2 Tbsp.   **Garlic Powder**

2 Tbsp.   **Paprika**

1 Tbsp.   **Sea Salt**

2 Tsp.	Cayenne Pepper
1 Tbsp.	Thyme
1 Tbsp.	Black Pepper, Ground
1 Tbsp.	Cumin
1 Tbsp.	Lime Juice
2 Tbsp.	Extra Virgin Olive Oil

Instructions

Slice chicken breasts into thin strips. Mix together spices with lemon juice and add chicken to bowl and coat. Heat olive oil in skillet and brown chicken strips until done. Pour seasoning into pan and stir. Allow chicken to simmer for 5 to 10 minutes, stirring during cooking to prevent sticking. Serve in Flour taco size tortillas topped with pico de gallo salsa (recipe above).

Sides

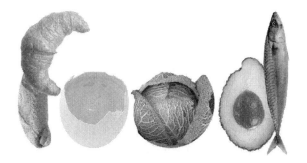

Side-dishes help balance your meal and compliment the protein that you're serving. It's important to choose foods from a variety of food groups and try to use foods from a variety of colors for the best nutrition. Careful spice choices can really bring out the flavors of your vegetables and add even more color to make your plates appealing.

Sweet Carrots with Fresh Marjoram

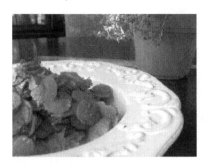

Carrots are always a sweet and fresh side dish filled with healthy nutrients. Dressed up with lemon juice, fresh marjoram, and garlic gives you a flavorful addition to any meal that is both healing and tasty.

Ingredients

2 lbs.	Carrots, Cut in Slices
1 Clove	Garlic, Peeled and Minced
3 Tbsp.	Extra Virgin Olive Oil
⅓ Tsp.	Sea Salt
¼ Tsp.	Black Pepper, Ground
1 Tsp.	Natural Sugar, Granulated
2 Tbsp.	Marjoram, Fresh and Chopped (Can substitute 1 Tbsp. Dried)

4 Tsp.	Lemon Juice

Instructions

Heat olive oil in skillet and saute carrots, sugar, and garlic. Lightly salt and pepper. Saute until carrots begin to soften. Sprinkle in marjoram and simmer gently with lid on pan for 5 to 6 minutes.

Remove cover from pan and turn heat up. Saute carrots until they begin to slightly brown. Remove from heat, sprinkle with lemon juice and serve immediately.

Roasted Red Potatoes with Rosemary

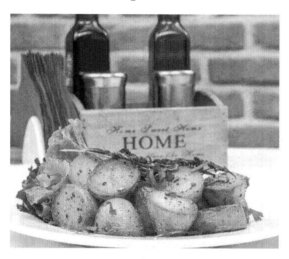

Red potatoes are a perfect pairing for meals spanning your entire day. You can toss these up with your eggs at breakfast, or enjoy them as a side for lunch or dinner. The rosemary gives you multiple benefits and a savory herb flavor for your potatoes.

Ingredients

10 to 12   **Red   Potatoes,   Peeled   or Unpeeled and halved**

2 Tbsp.   **Rosemary, Fresh/Minced**

2 Tbsp.   **Garlic, Fresh/Minced**

¼ c.	Extra Virgin Olive Oil
1 Tsp.	Sea Salt
¼ Tsp.	Black Pepper, Ground

Directions

Set oven temp to 400°F and preheat for 10 to 15 mins. Place halved potatoes in large bowl and toss with; salt, pepper, rosemary, garlic and olive oil. Turn potatoes out onto a baking sheet, making sure they are well separated. Bake in oven for 30 minutes, then turn with spatula. Allow to cook 30 minutes longer until crispy and brown. Serve immediately.

Spiced Rice

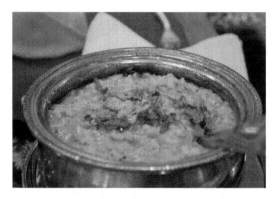

This tasty creation is infused with several of the spices known to help reduce gout symptoms and increase your body's ability to heal. This side-dish works well with a steamy bowl of lentils, tandoori chicken, or even your favorite tofu dish.

Ingredients

1 Pkg.	**Basmati Rice, 10-12 Ounces**
1	**Onion, Small/Chopped**
1 Clove	**Garlic, Peeled/Chopped**
1 Stick	**Butter**
1 Can	**Vegetable Broth**

½ Tsp.	Coriander Seeds
1 Stick	Cinnamon
1 Tsp.	Cumin Seeds
4-5 Pods	Cardamom
1 Tsp.	Turmeric
½ Tsp.	Mustard Seeds, Black
2	Bay Leaves
½ Tsp.	Sea Salt
¼ Tsp.	Black Pepper, Ground

Instructions

Grind coriander seeds to powder. Grind cardamom until just crushed. Crush cinnamon sticks. Grind cumin seeds. This all needs to be done separately, then mix together. You can use a mortar and pestle or electric grinder.

Take ½ stick of butter and melt in a pan. Saute the garlic and onion, then add turmeric and mustard seed to pan. Saute for 2 minutes, then add all spices from grinder mixture. Stir for another 2 minutes.

Add rice to pan and coat. Pour in broth, add salt and pepper and bring to a boil. Reduce heat and cover, allowing to simmer 15 to 20 minutes until broth is absorbed into rice. When finished, remove from heat.

Cut ½ stick of butter into cubes and add to rice. Allow it to melt into rice then fluff with a fork. Do not overstir to avoid breaking down rice. Cover with lid and allow to steep another 5 minutes with heat off. Top with bay leaves. Remind those eating to pull out any uncrushed cinnamon.

Breakfast

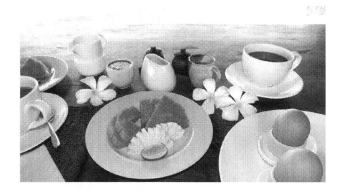

It has always been said that, "breakfast is the most important meal of the day!" Your body has just come off a 6 to 8 hour fast and needs fuel to start the day. What better way to fuel your body with energy to heal from gout, and get the benefits of spices for gout relief. Here are some quick and easy ideas to give your body a good start.

Fruited Oatmeal with Cinnamon and Flax

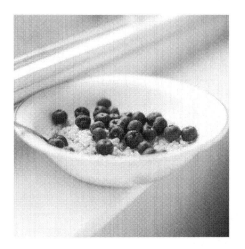

Oatmeal is a basic staple that is quick and easy for busy mornings. You can top it with basically any fruit you like. It's what is in the oatmeal that will have the most impact on your health. Add in a sprinkle of flax for antioxidants, and cinnamon for anti-inflammatory action. Plus, oatmeal is high in fiber and keeps you full until lunchtime.

Ingredients

1 c.	Steel Cut Oats
2 c.	Spring Water
¼ c.	Milk
½ Tsp.	Sea Salt
½ Tsp.	Cinnamon
1 Tbsp.	Flax Seeds, Ground to open hulls
½ c.	Fruit of your choice

Instructions

Bring water and salt to boil. Add oatmeal and milk. Allow to simmer 5 minutes if regular oats and 3 minutes if quick cook type. Turn off heat, and stir in Cinnamon and flax seeds and cover. Allow to steep another 3 to 5 minutes. Place oatmeal in bowl and top with your choice of; berries, bananas, apples, peaches, or any other fruit you like.

Spiced Wheat Pancakes

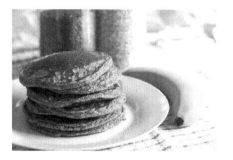

You won't even be able to tell the difference between this "healthier" version of pancakes using whole wheat flour, and the usual buttermilk pancakes with white flour. They still come out just as light and fluffy, with the added benefit of ground cloves, and cinnamon for your gout symptoms. You can even make a batch of this batter and store it in an airtight container in your fridge for up to 3 days.

Ingredients

2 c.	**Wheat Flour**
1 Tbsp.	**Baking Powder**
½ Tsp.	**Sea Salt**
½ Tsp.	**Ground Clove**
1 Tsp.	**Cinnamon**

¼ Tsp.	Nutmeg
3	Eggs, Large
2 c.	Buttermilk
½ Stick	Butter, Melted
1 Tbsp.	Sugar

Instructions

Sift together; flour, baking powder, salt, sugar, and spices in a large bowl and set aside. Melt butter in small bowl and set aside. In medium bowl whisk together; buttermilk, and eggs. Pour buttermilk mixture into large bowl with flour mixture and add melted butter. Stir gently just until batter is wet and leave some lumps. Do not overmix. Drop onto heated greased griddle and allow bubbles to form in batter before turning. Cook about 3 minutes on each side and serve right away with warm maple syrup or top with fruit.

Eggs Ranchero with Rosemary Toast

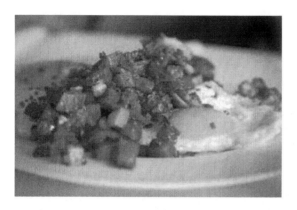

Eggs ranchero is essentially just fried eggs with a heap of salsa on top. This gives you the benefit of fresh vegetables, cilantro, and the healthy protein from eggs. Adding a piece of rosemary sourdough bread gives you something to mop up that yolk, and the healing benefits of rosemary.

Ingredients

2	Eggs, Large
¼ c.	Pico de Gallo Salsa (Recipe Above)
¼ Tsp.	Sea Salt
¼ Tsp.	Black Pepper, Ground
1 Tbsp.	Extra Virgin Olive OIl

2 Slices	Sourdough Bread
½ Tsp.	Rosemary, Crushed
2 Pats	Butter

Instructions

Heat oven to 325 degrees. Butter both sides of bread and sprinkle on Rosemary. Place on baking sheet in oven. Heat olive oil in skillet and crack in eggs. Fry to desired doneness and slide onto plate. Top with salsa. Check toast and remove from oven when brown on both sides, about 5 minutes. You may need to flip bread at about 3 minutes. Remove toast from oven, place on plate and garnish plate with fresh fruit if you like.

Peppermint Lemon Balm Tea and Muffins

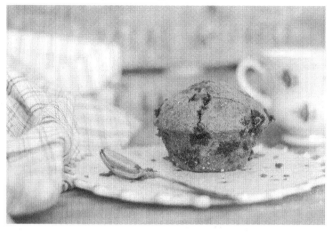

If you don't have time for a cooked breakfast, a quick alternative would be a tea containing herbs to relieve gout symptoms and a muffin. This helps fill your stomach and have some relief on board to start your day. The peppermint has properties that can help lower uric acid levels. Lemon balm is both an anti-inflammatory and has diuretic properties that helps to flush out toxins like, uric acid.

To make Tea:

Take 2 tablespoons of fresh peppermint and 2 Tablespoons dried lemon balm and add to small teapot. Pour 2 cups boiling water over and allow to steep for 5 to 10 minutes. Makes 2 cups of tea.

Enjoy with your favorite muffins either homemade or bakery fresh.

Belgian Waffles with Lavender Cream and Berries

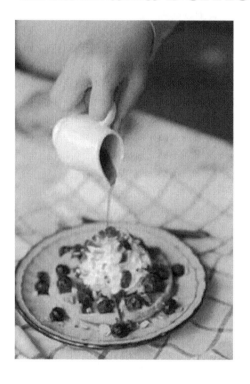

Waffles are always a hit at breakfast. They are sweet and filled with energizing carbs to refuel your body. Infusing cream with lavender can help you reduce gout symptoms and makes a beautiful presentation when topped with fresh fruit.

Waffle Ingredients

2 c.	Flour
½ Tsp.	Sea Salt, Fine
4 Tsp.	Baking Powder
¼ c.	Raw Sugar, Granulated
2 c.	Milk
½ c.	Oil
2 Large	Eggs, Separated

Instructions

Sift together; flour, baking soda, and salt. Add in sugar. In a separate bowl, whisk together egg yolks and milk. Pour in oil and stir. In another bowl, beat the egg whites until they form stiff peaks.

Pour milk mixture into flour mixture and stir. Fold egg whites into mix. Spray waffle iron with cooking spray and cook waffle batter ⅛ to ¼ cup at a time until brown. Top with lavender whipped cream (recipe below) and fresh fruit. You can also use real maple syrup with or without the cream.

Lavender Whipped Cream

This dreamy whipped topping can be used on waffles, pancakes, or even desserts. It has a slight hint of fragrant lavender and lightly sweet.

Ingredients

1 c.   **Heavy Whipping Cream**

1 c.   **Berries   (blueberries,   raspberries, strawberries, etc.)**

2 Tbsp.   **Sugar, Superfine**

2 Tsp.   **Lavender, Dried and Crushed with mortar and pestle**

Instructions

Add heavy cream and lavender to saucepan and simmer lightly for 2 to 3 minutes. Pour through strainer and toss lavender. Place bowl in fridge and chill until cold. Pour into a cold metal or glass bowl and whip with mixer until peaks form. Add sugar a little a a time and beat. Place back into fridge and chill before use. (Best made the night before)

Desserts

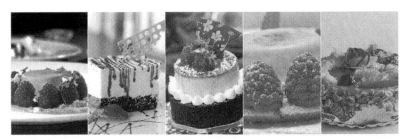

Desserts aren't always sinful, as a matter of fact, they can be quite healthy if the right ingredients are used. These tasty treats are a great way to end your meal and give your body a boost of gout fighting nutrients.

Snickerdoodles

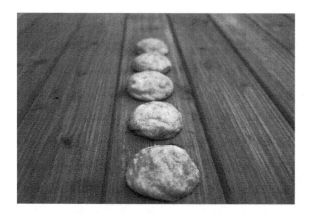

These warm cookies are always a hit and easy to make. They combine a simple sugar cookie recipe and coated with cinnamon sugar. You can make the basic dough the night before and chill for best baking results. A little patience and you get the perfect chewy inside and crispy outside. The cinnamon will help benefit gout symptoms and satisfy sweet cravings!

Ingredients

2 ½ c.	**Flour**
1 ½ c.	**Raw Sugar, Granulated**
1 Tsp.	**Baking Soda**
¼ Tsp.	**Sea Salt, Fine**
2 Tsp.	**Cream of Tartar**

2 Tbsp.	Sugar, Granulated (Set Aside for Topping)
1 Tbsp.	Cinnamon
1 c.	Butter
2 Large	Eggs
1 Tbsp.	Vanilla Extract

Instructions

Heat oven to 350 degrees. In large bowl, sift together; flour, cream of tartar, baking soda, and salt. In separate bowl; cream butter, sugar, vanilla, and eggs. Blend all ingredients together and turn out onto plastic wrap. Wrap tightly and place in fridge for up to 2 hours. In large zip bag, mix together sugar and cinnamon. Remove dough from fridge and form into 1 to 2 inch balls. Place in zip bag and shake to coat with cinnamon mixture. Place on cookie sheet and bake 8 to 10 minutes until lightly browned.

Peppermint White Chocolate Mousse

1 ½ c.   Heavy Cream

12 oz.   White Chocolate Chips, Semi-Sweet

½ Tsp.   Peppermint Extract

2 Tbsp.   Peppermint Candy, Crushed

Instructions

Place ¾ of the heavy cream in a saucepan and heat slowly while whisking. Do not boil. Turn off heat when hot and pour in chocolate chips. Stir well until all chips are melted. Add peppermint extract and stir.

Cool in fridge until completely cooled. In a separate bowl, beat remainder of heavy cream until stiff peaks form. Take cooled chocolate mixture from fridge and stir into beaten cream very gently. Spoon into ramekins and top with crushed candies.

Carrot Cake with Lavender Cream Cheese Frosting

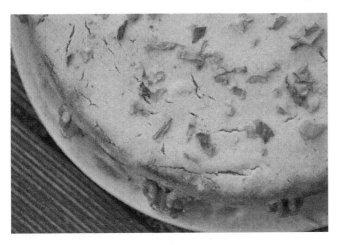

Carrot cake is always a favorite for dessert. This version incorporates both cinnamon and lavender for two gout relieving ingredients and doesn't skimp on deliciousness! Make the frosting up the night before so the lavender oils can soak in nicely. Organic ingredients will give your cake a "fresh from the garden" taste to please your tastebuds.

Cake Ingredients

2 c.	Organic Cake Flour/or All Purpose Flour
1 c.	Organic Raw Sugar
2 c.	Carrots, Peeled/Grated/Water Squeezed Out
2 Tsp.	Baking Soda
1 Tsp.	Baking Powder
½ Tsp.	Sea Salt
2 Tsp.	Cinnamon, Ground
½ Tsp.	Nutmeg, Ground
½ Tsp.	Lavender, Dried
1 Tbsp.	Orange Zest
2 Large	Eggs, Cage-Free Organic
¾ c.	Extra Virgin Olive Oil
2 Tsp.	Organic Vanilla Extract

(½ c. Chopped Walnuts if desired)

Cake Instructions

Heat oven to 350 degrees. Grease 4 cake pans (about 5") or 2 eight inch pans. Sift together; flour, baking soda, baking powder, salt, and spices. Cream together; eggs, sugar and vanilla. Stir in vanilla and oil and mix into flour mixture. Make sure carrots are well-drained by pushing into strainer and squeezing in towels. Stir in carrots and lavender.

Pour batter into pans and bake 20 to 30 minutes until toothpick comes out clean in center. Cool on racks and frost with frosting below.

Frosting Ingredients

3 Tbsp.	Butter, Organic/Unsalted
3 oz.	Cream Cheese
2 c.	Powdered Sugar, Organic
2 Tsp.	Vanilla Extract, Organic
2 Tbsp.	Lavender, Dried/Crushed

Instructions

Soften butter and cream cheese to room temperature while mixing and baking cake. Place into mixing bowl and blend with vanilla until smooth. Mix in powdered sugar a few tablespoons at a time. Sprinkle in lavender and mix well. Spread on cakes when cool. You can save a few sprigs of fresh lavender with purple flowers to garnish the cake if you like.

Beverages

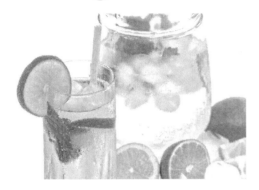

A warm cup of tea on a rainy day or a cool drink on a hot day can refresh you and help with your gout symptoms. You can take a number of beverages and add spices that help relieve gout symptoms. The possibilities are endless, but here are a few to help you get started.

Cinnamon Licorice Tea

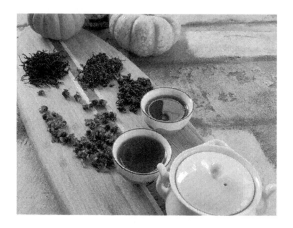

Make sure you ask your doctor before consuming licorice, especially if you have high blood pressure

Cinnamon licorice tea can be taken either hot or cold and has two great spices for gout relief. Brew this up and keep it in your fridge to take up to 2 cups a day.

Ingredients

1 Tbsp.   **Green or Black Tea**

1 Tbsp.   **Licorice, Ground**

1 Tsp.   **Cinnamon, Crushed**

Instructions

Take tea, licorice and cinnamon and mix together. Place in tea bag or strainer and pour one cup of boiling water over. Steep for 5 minutes and remove tea. Stir in honey to taste, if you like. Drink one to two cups daily.

Peppermint Iced Tea

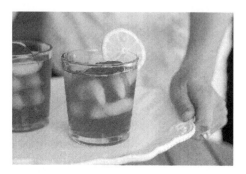

Peppermint iced tea is a refreshing drink for any kind of day whether hot or even rainy. The peppermint can relieve your gout symptoms and give your body a cool sensation that soothes pain. You can even take some of the brewed tea and use it as a compress on sore joints.

Ingredients

6 Tbsp.	**Peppermint Leaves, Fresh or Dried**
2 Sprigs	**Peppermint, Fresh**
6 c.	**Boiling Water**
3 c.	**Ice**

Instructions

Place tea in saucepan and add 6 cups boiling water. Cover pan and allow to steep for 10 to 15 minutes. Remove lid and cool down with peppermint in pan. Strain into 2 quart pitcher over ice cubes. Top with sprigs of peppermint. Serve in iced glasses.

Clove Tea

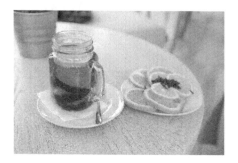

Cloves are a strong and spicy herb that actually make delicious herbal tea. You won't have to use as much as other herbs or steep it as long to get the flavor. It works well hot or cold and gives relief to gout pain, while quenching your thirst.

Ingredients

1 Tsp.   **Clove, Ground**

1 c.   **Boiling Water**

2-3 Slices   **Orange**

Instructions

Stick to about 1 teaspoon of clove or the tea may come out too potent. You can adjust the amount to your taste after you try it a few times. Take the clove and place in tea bag or strainer. Pour boiling water over tea and steep for about 5 minutes or to your taste. Remove tea and garnish with orange slices.

Gout 10 day Meal Plan

Working in spices to your weekly meal plan can help you get the most from the foods you eat while you are healing from gout. It can also help you maintain your ability to fight off and prevent future gout attacks.

All you really need to do is take note of the above spices that can help you. Add a sprinkle of cinnamon to your toast or oatmeal everyday, or drop some lemon balm into your smoothie. You can also end your meal with a cup of hot clove tea.

The recipes above will get you started, but try to find new recipes to give yourself some variety. This way, you are eating healthy meals that help combat inflammation, pain, and elevated uric acid level.

Breakfast – Lunch - Dinner

Day 1   Oatmeal with Cinnamon

Fresh Blueberries

Toast   Curried pumpkin carrot soup

Chicken Salad Sandwich Glazed Ham with Clove

Sweet Carrots with Fresh Marjoram

Carrot Cake with Lavender Cream Cheese Frosting

Day 2   Eggs Ranchero with Pico de Gallo
Toast   Ham Sandwich
Pickled Cucumber Salad
Grilled Steak
Pickled Cucumber Salad

Day 3   Spiced Wheat Pancakes

Sausage   Spring Mix Greens

with Fennel Bulb

Grilled Chicken Breast Pork

Chops with Chopped Basil and

Peaches

Rice or Potato

Day 4   Scrambled Eggs Peppermint Lemon Balm Tea and a muffin   Pork Chops with Chopped Basil and Peaches Stinging Nettle Pesto over Pasta Baguette

Day 5   Cold Cereal
Toast
Clove Tea Stinging Nettle Pesto over Pasta
Green Salad   Chicken Tacos with Pico de Gallo

Day 6   Belgian Waffles with Lavender Cream and Berries

Ham Slice Chicken Tacos with Pico de Gallo

Grilled Salmon

Roasted Red Potatoes with Rosemary

Day 7   Fruited Oatmeal with Cinnamon and Flax

Fried egg (optional)

Toast   Spring Mix Greens with Fennel Bulb topped with Grilled Salmon

Curried pumpkin carrot soup

Baguette

Snickerdoodles

Day 8   Scrambled Eggs with Pico de Gallo

Fresh Strawberries

Toast

Fresh Fruit   Spring Mix Greens with Fennel Bulb

Grilled Chicken Breast   Coriander Chicken

Spiced Rice

Peppermint White Chocolate Mousse

Day 9　Cinnamon Licorice Tea

Muffin of Choice　Coriander

Chicken

Green Salad

Fresh Fruit Pork Chops with

Chopped Basil and Peaches

Sweet Carrots with Fresh

Marjoram

Day 10 Egg Sandwich on Rosemary Toast

Peppermint Tea Curried pumpkin carrot soup Baguette Pizza Night!

Peppermint White Chocolate Mousse

This meal plan is designed to make some things in larger batches and use some meals for leftover lunches. This helps you save time and get the most out of your meals. Make up large batches of salsa for marinades, toppings and snacking with chips. Mousse, cookies and cakes will all keep for up to two weeks if wrapped and stored properly.

You can also mix and match this menu with your own personal weekly menu to give you more meal options. You can even experiment with the spices above in your own favorite dishes.

Try to include a variety of beverages to help balance your diet. Good ideas include:

- Flax Milk
- Juices (cranberry, orange, grapefruit, and apple)
- Spring Water
- Herbal Tea
- Mineral Water
- Almond or Rice Milks
- Coconut Water

Try to avoid caffeinated beverages like coffee and caramel colored soda, they can increase the risk of kidney stones. To help flush uric acid, increase your fluid intake. Water is always best and you should try to get at least 2 liters a day.

Lifestyle Changes For Preventing Gout

Along with a healthy diet incorporating the spices listed above, there are several lifestyle changes you can do to help you recover from gout and prevent future flares. Try these practices every day, and exercise as much as you can tolerate without too much pain. Here are some good lifestyle changes for living with gout:

Increase Fluid Intake. It is recommended that you try to drink at least 2 liters of water daily, more or less depending on your doctor's recommendations. A good way to measure out water intake, is to clean out a 2 liter soda bottle and fill it for the day. If you drink it all you can always refill it. Try to use filtered or spring water if you can. Keep a portable water bottle with you at all times during the day and sip often. If you take water in the car, try to use a glass or metal water bottle.

Balance Your Diet. In addition to the recipes and meal plan above, try to include plenty of; fresh vegetables, fresh fruits, whole grains, lean proteins, healthy fats, and a few servings of calcium foods daily. Reduce your intake of starchy carbohydrates, sugar, and high fructose corn syrup. Try switching to raw unrefined sugar and/or honey.

Reduce or Avoid Alcohol. Alcohol can increase gout symptoms, elevate uric acid levels, and increase the risk of kidney stones. Beer is especially high in purines that can raise your uric acid levels. New studies show that beer should be avoided, but less than two glasses of wine daily may be safe. Other spirits may increase the risk of gout. If you drink more than two alcoholic beverages daily, it is important to discuss this with your doctor and get help if you need it.

Focus on Healthy Fats. Not all fats are bad. Try to get healthy fats from; avocado, extra virgin olive oil, nuts, and coconut oil. Reduce your intake of; animal fats, corn oil, margarine, trans and saturated fats, and shortening. This will help speed up weight loss and has protective benefits to your cardiovascular system, which can indirectly be affected by gout.

Try To Lose Excess Weight. Obesity and extra weight not only increases your risk of gout, but can worsen acute flares. In the meal plan above, you can always skip desserts and add more leafy greens to your diet, if needed. Being overweight with gout puts excess strain on your hips, knees, and feet, and can make walking very difficult. Eating a diet high in foods that cause weight gain may be high in purines and raise your uric acid levels. Getting on a healthy gout diet, even if you are only at risk may reduce your chances of an acute flare.

Avoid Purine Foods. Avoid foods that are high in purines. Purines convert into uric acid, this causes the uric acid crystals that irritate the joints during a gout flare. Some high purine foods include:

- Liver, Brain, Kidney, and other organ meat
- Mackerel, Anchovy, Mussels, Fish Eggs, Sardines, and Scallops (Salmon is a good seafood if eaten in moderation)
- Gravy, Cream Sauces, Cheese Sauce
- Rich Foods (foods made with meat fats)
- Cured Meats (Bacon, lunch meats, hot dogs, pork chops, cured ham)
- Lamb
- Venison, Bison, Moose Meat
- Asparagus (Mild Risk)
- Spinach (Mild Risk)

Naturally, you won't want to completely avoid some foods. If they are a mild or low-risk food, you may want to just reduce your consumption.

Increase Vitamin C Intake. While it has been shown in recent studies that vitamin C may not have any benefits in reducing uric acid levels as once thought, it may help with gout prevention. If you are at risk for gout, try to get more than 250 mg and 1500 mg of vitamin C daily from foods like; oranges, kiwi, broccoli, and other citrus fruits. One thing that citric acid may help with is reducing the build-up of crystal forming materials in the kidneys during a gout flare.

Increase Potassium Intake. Foods high in potassium may also help stop uric acid crystals from forming in the urine. Increasing potassium foods like; oranges and orange juice, bananas, potatoes, and lima beans. The type of potassium that can help reduce uric acid crystals in urine is either citrate or maleate. You can also ask your doctor about an over-the-counter supplement if he or she thinks you may need it.

Try Lemon Juice Daily. A daily squeeze of lemon in your water can be a very powerful antioxidant. This can help neutralize the uric acid that runs through the kidneys, helping it pass from the body more effectively. Lemon juice starts cleaning out the blood that runs through your liver removing toxins there and then on to the kidneys. Just use caution if you have any digestive disorders or any form of acidosis.

Use Low-Fat Dairy Products or Dairy Alternatives. The lower in fat your dairy products, the better. High fat dairy products may contain higher purine levels. Try to use low-fat or skim milk and cheese. If you can, try to switch to dairy alternatives. Just avoid soy products, they tend to raise uric acid levels. Good alternatives include; almond milk, flax milk, or coconut milk. There are also some delicious vegan cheeses made from nuts.

Exercise 3 Times A Week. During an acute flare, you may be stuck in bed for a week or even two. After the flare subsides, begin walking at a moderate pace a few times a week, as tolerated with your doctor's okay. You can also try some gentle yoga stretches when you're feeling better and light weight bearing exercises. This will help you lose any excess weight and increase the strength of your muscles around the affected joints.

If you have had a particularly severe gout flare, your doctor may recommend physical therapy to start. They can work with you to gently get your strength back and teach you exercises to use at home. You can also talk to your doctor about enrolling in a "gentle yoga" class designed for people with arthritis. While powerful advanced type yoga may overstretch the joints, gentle yoga may actually help improve stability.

Double Check Drug Interactions. Most importantly, when using any complementary or alternative medicine approaches with gout, always check for drug/herb interactions with your doctor. When you go for your doctor visits, take a list of things you are taking and eating with you so your doctor can compare them for interactions. It is also a good idea to let your pharmacy know, as well. Some spices and herbal remedies may interact with other health conditions or medications. For instance; omega-3 supplements and garlic can also have blood thinning effects and may not be appropriate if you are on blood thinning medications. Likewise, if you are on a blood thinner, some foods are high in vitamin K and may counteract the blood thinner. While certain drugs may be used for other health conditions, they may be affected by home remedies for gout. The good news is most spices that you use in cooking are considered generally safe when used in moderation.

Conclusion

Cooking with spices for gout relief can be a very healthy complement to your gout treatment plan. Meals can be planned for one person, two people, or an entire family and they are tasty enough for everyone to enjoy. Plus, you get the benefits of helping your body reduce uric acid levels, lower inflammation and feel better fast!

Always consult your doctor for your individual needs. This book is not intended to be a substitute for the medical advice of a licensed physician. The reader should consult with their doctor in any matters relating to his/her health.

We thank you, and value your comments, and reviews for this book. Please share your experience with others, so they may benefit from your knowledge on the subject. Your experiences, and thoughts, can help benefit those struggling, more than you could possibly imagine. Placing your ideas, and experiences in the review section of this book, will make it seen by others, who will benefit from your help. 5 minutes of your time, can help change someone's life for the better. Thank you.

GOUT

Prevention

a metabolic disorder
unic acid

the deposition and accumulation
of salts in the joint

GOUT

inflammation and pain
in the small joints

Geoff Andersen

With Meal Plan &
Gout Recipes

Made in the USA
San Bernardino, CA
15 May 2020